Advance Prais
Psychodynamic Psychopharmacology

"Mintz's *Psychodynamic Psychopharmacology: Caring for the Treatment-Resistant Patient* turns the problem of treatment resistance on its head—it's not caused by an inadequate pill; it arises from the complexity of the patient. Master psychopharmacologists are usually master psychotherapists in disguise, and this systematic discussion of the personal, relational, emotional, and symbolic aspects of medication treatment provides both an erudite understanding of these factors and wonderful practical advice about how to handle them."

—*Richard F. Summers, M.D., Clinical Professor of Psychiatry and Senior Residency Advisor, Perelman School of Medicine of the University of Pennsylvania*

"David Mintz, an award-winning educator and experienced clinician, creates a road map to help us understand and navigate treatment resistance, inspired by the biopsychosocial model and patient-centered medicine, approaches that optimize care and prevent burnout and moral injury among physicians. This book summarizes evidence-based research addressing the relevance of placebo and nocebo effects in all clinical practice, the meaning of medication, and factors that positively or adversely affect the therapeutic alliance and doctor–patient interactions. Mintz also provides manualized guidelines for the practice of psychopharmacology in challenging clinical situations where multimorbidities, unconscious conflicts, negative attitudes, avoidant attachments, ambivalence, and treatment nonadherence interfere with adequate clinical care. This accessible book will be helpful to all psychiatric trainees and their supervisors, who will invariably face the challenges of treatment resistance in everyday practice."

—*César A. Alfonso, M.D., Clinical Professor of Psychiatry at Columbia University, Editor of Psychodynamic Psychiatry, and Chair of the Section on Psychotherapy of the World Psychiatric Association.*

"Dr. David Mintz has done a great service in this excellent book for those who prescribe psychiatric medications: he has provided an important approach to optimizing treatment outcomes by integrating pharmacotherapy with a psychodynamically-informed perspective that enhances therapeutic factors for the patient and the doctor–patient encounter. Through clinical examples and literature review, he has defined what many clinicians have learned through experience but were not taught as part of their psychopharmacology education. The interpersonal context of the prescribing relationship between prescriber and patient may have deep psychodynamic meaning to many patients. Understanding these factors (such as transference to parental figures) can enhance the adherence and effectiveness of treatments. I recommend this book for all psychopharmacology prescribers."

—*Carl Salzman, M.D., Professor of Psychiatry, Harvard Medical School*

"David Mintz and colleagues have written an invaluable book for those who prescribe psychotropic medications. With rich theoretical background, vivid case examples, and practical clinical advice, they offer prescribers a way to elicit and address patient concerns that can strengthen the doctor–patient alliance and in this way improve the patient experience with medication use. This is a book for clinicians at all levels of experience and should be assigned reading for psychiatrists in training."

—*Robert J. Waldinger, M.D.*

"If you are at an impasse with your patients despite optimal psychopharmacology, in all likelihood the problem is not with the biology but with the powerful psychology of the person and the therapist. *Psychodynamic Psychopharmacology* provides a road map for overcoming the impasse and achieving positive outcomes. This is a must-read for all psychiatrists in today's world of managed care and time-limited treatment."

—*Steven S. Sharfstein, M.D., President Emeritus, Sheppard Pratt Health System, and Past President, American Psychiatric Association*

"David Mintz's new book broadens the scope of the current reductionist model in biological psychiatry by introducing prescribers to the relational dimension of psychopharmacology provision, which often spells the difference between successful and failed treatments. Based on his team's extensive experience with treatment-resistant patients at the Austen Riggs Center, Dr. Mintz's state-of-the-art manual systematically reviews subjective and intersubjective factors contributing to psychopharmacological treatment outcomes that complement the current biomedical treatment algorithms.

The newly formulated field of psychodynamic psychopharmacology shifts clinical attention from the prevalent symptomatic treatment approach to evidence-based principles of care, which include the person of our patient, the meaning of the treatment, and the relational dimension of the treatment provision. The book chapters systematically review the rationale and evidence for psychodynamic psychopharmacology and address a range of topics, including medication resistance, patient autonomy, the attachment dimension behind transference reenactments in the treatment setting, and the importance of paying attention to the clinician's countertransference response. Part 3 provides a step-by-step treatment manual with relevant clinical vignettes that would benefit both beginning and seasoned practitioners. I would highly recommend this book as an indispensable resource for every psychiatric residency program and every prescribing clinician."

— *Yakov Shapiro, M.D., Clinical Professor and Psychotherapy Supervisor, Department of Psychiatry, University of Alberta, and Clinical Director, Integrated Psychotherapy/Psychopharmacology Service (IPPS), Edmonton, Canada*

"A compelling case for bridging the mind-body divide in psychiatry through a psychodynamic lens. Dr. Mintz outlines a way forward that improves outcomes for patient and practitioner. This is truly patient-centered, affirming care."

—*Kathryn Kieran, PMHNP-BC, Psychiatric Mental Health Nurse Practitioner, McLean Hospital*

"*Psychodynamic Psychopharmacology* is the book and approach we need for appreciating the treatment-resistant patient. Mintz writes with decades of clinical experience and builds upon a century of evidence-based research to understand treatment resistance, and patients experiencing treatment resistance, differently. Mintz teaches us how to seek understanding of the people we meet as patients and allows the unconscious to become conscious: the way forward for psychiatry is to renew the therapeutic alliance."

> —*Abraham M. Nussbaum, M.D., MTS, DFAPA, Chief Education Officer, Denver Health, and Associate Professor of Psychiatry, University of Colorado School of Medicine*

"*Psychodynamic Psychopharmacology* is a welcome book with a crucial message. Our patients are more than bundles of molecules and receptors; they come to us with a suitcase full of life experiences that affect their attitudes and their ability to collaborate in treatment of any kind. Illness-driven behavior is not just willful oppositionalism. Read this book to be reminded of the rich, but often torn, fabric of a human life and the need to know all about it. Then get out your prescription pad."

> —*John M. Oldham, M.D., Distinguished Emeritus Professor, Menninger Department of Psychiatry and Behavioral Sciences, Baylor College of Medicine*

"Following the dictates of evidence-based prescribing remains problematic in all of medicine. What about the person receiving the treatment, the prescriber, and their relationship? David Mintz beautifully demonstrates the clinical value of integrating each of these and other variables into the treatment process."

> —*Bernard D. Beitman, M.D., Visiting Professor, Department of Psychiatry and Behavioral Sciences, University of Virginia, and Founding Director, The Coincidence Project*

Psychodynamic Psychopharmacology

Caring for the Treatment-Resistant Patient

Psychodynamic Psychopharmacology

Caring for the Treatment-Resistant Patient

By
David Mintz, M.D., DFAPA

The Austen Riggs Center,
Stockbridge, Massachusetts

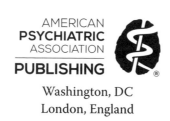

AMERICAN
PSYCHIATRIC
ASSOCIATION
PUBLISHING

Washington, DC
London, England

If you wish to buy 50 or more copies of the same title, visit www.appi.org/specialdiscounts for more information.

Copyright © 2022 American Psychiatric Association Publishing

ALL RIGHTS RESERVED

First Edition

Manufactured in the United States of America on acid-free paper
26 25 24 23 22   5 4 3 2 1

American Psychiatric Association Publishing
800 Maine Avenue SW, Suite 900
Washington, DC 20024-2812 www.appi.org

Library of Congress Cataloging-in-Publication Data

Names: Mintz, David L. author. | American Psychiatric Association Publishing, issuing body.
Title: Psychodynamic psychopharmacology : caring for the treatment-resistant patient / by David Mintz.
Description: First edition. | Washington, DC : American Psychiatric Association Publishing, [2022] | Includes bibliographical references and index.
Identifiers: LCCN 2021050419 (print) | LCCN 2021050420 (ebook) | ISBN 9781615371525 (paperback) | ISBN 9781615374007 (ebook)
Subjects: MESH: Mental Disorders--drug therapy | Psychotropic Drugs—therapeutic use | Treatment Refusal—psychology | Physician–Patient Relations
Classification: LCC RM315 (print) | LCC RM315 (ebook) | NLM WM 402 | DDC 615.7/88—dc23/eng/20211209
LC record available at https://lccn.loc.gov/2021050419
LC ebook record available at https://lccn.loc.gov/2021050420

British Library Cataloguing in Publication Data

A CIP record is available from the British Library.

Contents

Part III
The Manual of Psychodynamic Psychopharmacology

Appendixes

Preface

For much of the past century, Western psychiatry was dominated by psychoanalysis. Although Freud himself was optimistic about future biomedical treatments (Freud 1926/1959, 1940[1938]/1964; Simmel 1937), this did not prevent divisions within psychiatry in which somatic treatments were denigrated as addressing patients' symptoms but failing to achieve a deeper cure. When biomedical psychiatry came into ascendance in the last quarter of the 20th century, psychoanalysis received the same treatment in return. Under the banner of evidence-based medicine, much of the accumulated wisdom of psychoanalysis was disparaged as groundless, especially because psychodynamic psychiatry was late to the game in accumulating an evidence base (McWilliams 2013). Unfortunately, despite our mushrooming understanding of neuroscience and increasing focus on evidence-based treatments, there is little indication that outcomes are substantially improved. Rather, treatment resistance is increasingly recognized as a major issue in psychiatry.

One likely source of the epidemic of psychiatric treatment resistance is the general neglect of psychodynamic and psychosocial factors in psychiatry, beginning with the biomedical tilt in psychiatry at the end of the 20th century (Plakun 2006). The focus on "evidence" in psychiatric research and the psychiatric literature has meant a focus on neuroscientific evidence and a general neglect of psychosocial factors in prescribing. It has also led to a disparagement of viewpoints that draw from the accumulated wisdom of psychoanalysis (Plakun 2012). Consequently, psychosocial evidence bases have, in recent years, been largely neglected by academic psychiatry (Mintz and Flynn 2012), including those that apply to psychopharmacology.

Economic and political factors in medicine have reshaped the doctor–patient relationship in ways that often minimize the impact of potentially mutative psychosocial factors. Models of compensation by third-party payers have favored the development of "15-minute med checks," in which the focus is more on medications and symptoms and less on the person *with* the symptoms. The increasing use of symptom checklists to evaluate patients' response to medications has further promoted an "illness-centered" perspective that fails to capitalize on the potential benefits of a patient-centered perspective. In addition, the introduction of the electronic medical record often has the effect of focusing prescribers on their digital device rather than on their patient, further chipping away at the potential health benefits of a more person-centered doctor–patient relationship. These effects not only occurred at the level of the individual relationship of doctors and patients but also began to tarnish the public perception of psychiatry, so that psychiatrists often began treatments from a position of substantial mistrust. For example, a 2009 Gallup Poll (Jones and Saad 2011) revealed that only 33% of Americans believed psychiatrists adhere to "high" or "very high" ethical standards. Alarmingly, this put them on par with bankers, even after the financial crisis of 2008, and significantly lower than nurses (83%) and medical doctors in general (65%).

Beginning in the early 2000s, the National Institute of Mental Health (NIMH) sought to address the problem of psychiatric treatment resistance by focusing on biological correlates of psychiatric illness while minimizing the focus on psychosocial factors. Although the goal was to identify new targets for biomedical treatment that would yield better outcomes, the effect of this myopic focus was to ignore research that could benefit patients almost immediately (e.g., by optimizing factors in the working relationship) while supporting research that would not likely benefit patients for a generation. As Plakun (2017) noted, "It is our patients who are left to suffer, while clinging to hope that the promised big breakthrough of brain and gene research is just around the corner, when it is still likely decades away" (p. 132). With the development of the Research Domain Criteria focusing on neurobiological mechanisms of psychiatric illness, what little funding was left essentially disappeared for studies examining aspects of the prescribing process, contributions of patient psychology to pharmacological treatment outcomes, or other psychosocial aspects of care directly affecting outcomes (Plakun 2017). Given what we are learning about the role of nonpharmacological factors in shaping pharmacological treatment outcomes, it is perhaps not surprising that, toward the end of his tenure, NIMH Director Thomas Insel concluded that "the unfortunate reality is that current medications help too few people to get better and very few people to get well" (Insel 2009, p. 704).

At the Austen Riggs Center we routinely treat patients who have failed to respond adequately to multiple pharmacological treatments, psychotherapies, and hospitalizations. Austen Riggs is a fully open psychoanalytic hospital with the explicit mission of understanding and treating patients who have been labeled "treatment resistant." The emphasis is on replacing external controls (e.g., locked doors, privilege systems) with highly engaged therapeutic relationships, a deeply questioning attitude about the meaning of symptoms and symptomatic behaviors, and a focus on patients' autonomous motivations and capacity to learn from experience (Plakun 2011). Our patients are not the "ideal patients" without comorbidities on whom most pharmacotherapeutic treatments are tested in placebo-controlled trials. Rather, our patients are like everyone else's patients: both diagnostically and psychologically complicated. On average, our patients carry six diagnoses, almost always with significant character pathology. More than half have histories of early adverse experiences, including physical and sexual trauma, significant losses, neglect, and serious family dysfunction. Approximately one-third of our patients meet criteria for PTSD.

Furthermore, it is quite common for our patients to have disturbed relationships with caregiving and authority that can undermine alliances or promote subtle perversions of the therapeutic task. They are often ambivalent about their illnesses because they have learned to extract covert gratification from the illness or its symptoms. As such, they may work, perhaps unconsciously, to undermine our therapeutic efforts. Frequently, these patients' early negative experiences with caregiving have been reaffirmed through subsequent engagements with the mental health system, deepening their ambivalence about treatment. Ultimately, these factors complicate, in profound but often covert ways, the healthy and effective use of medications. These are not patients who will typically respond to the algorithm that suggests a particular dosage increase or a change of medication because their resistance originates as much in their psyche as in their disturbed biology.

This book emerges out of two decades of work within the prescribing medical staff at the Austen Riggs Center to grapple with, understand, and address the problem of pharmacological treatment resistance. Our patients have been excellent teachers, revealing the myriad ways they can thwart our therapeutic aspirations, often with little conscious awareness of doing so. They show us, over and over, how we get it wrong and unwittingly become part of the treatment resistance. They have taught us that when treatment resistance is an aspect of the illness, there is usually a good reason for it. We have learned that to address pharmacological treatment resistance, we must understand and respect the patient's reasons for that resistance.

This book was born of a hope that an empirically testable model integrating an informed understanding of the psychodynamics of pharmacotherapy with evidence of the psychosocial aspects of prescribing would offer a credible antidote to the biological tilt that has developed in psychiatry in recent decades. With a combination of clinical wisdom, scalable techniques, and evidence, we hope to pave a way forward to a model of care that incorporates both biological and psychodynamic perspectives. We hope that the knowledge we have acquired over a century of learning at the Austen Riggs Center will not only benefit the hundred or so patients we treat yearly but also prove useful to prescribers with basic psychotherapeutic skills who work in more resource-limited environments with equally complicated patients.

References

Freud S: The question of lay analysis (1926), in Standard Edition of the Complete Psychological Works of Sigmund Freud, Vol 20. Translated and edited by Strachey J. London, Hogarth, 1959, pp 177–258

Freud S: An outline of psycho-analysis (1940[1938]), in Standard Edition of the Complete Psychological Works of Sigmund Freud, Vol 23. Translated and edited by Strachey J. London, Hogarth, 1964, pp 139–207

Insel TR: Disruptive insights in psychiatry: transforming a clinical discipline. J Clin Invest 119(4):700–705, 2009 19339761

Jones J, Saad L: Honesty and ethics Gallup poll. Gallup News Service, 2011. Available at: https://www.gallup.com/file/poll/151463/Honesty_Ethics_111212.pdf. Accessed August 25, 2019.

McWilliams N: Psychoanalysis and research: some reflections and opinions. Psychoanal Rev 100(6):919–945, 2013 24325186

Mintz DL, Flynn DF: How (not what) to prescribe: nonpharmacologic aspects of psychopharmacology. Psychiatr Clin North Am 35(1):143–163, 2012 22370496

Plakun EM: A view from Riggs—treatment resistance and patient authority: I. A psychodynamic perspective on treatment resistance. J Am Acad Psychoanal Dyn Psychiatry 34(2):349–366, 2006 16780414

Plakun EM: Introduction, in Treatment Resistance and Patient Authority: The Austen Riggs Reader. Edited by Plakun EM. New York, WW Norton, 2011, pp 1–5

Plakun EM: Treatment resistance and psychodynamic psychiatry: concepts psychiatry needs from psychoanalysis. Psychodyn Psychiatry 40(2):183–209, 2012 23006116

Plakun EM: Psychotherapy research and the NIMH: an either/or or both/and research agenda? J Psychiatr Pract 23(2):130–133, 2017 28291038

Simmel E: The psychoanalytic sanitarium and the psychoanalytic movement. Bull Menninger Clin 1(5):133–143, 1937

Acknowledgments

I acknowledge the contributions of my colleagues at the Austen Riggs Center, especially Barri Belnap, M.D., who sifted with me through everything we had learned at Riggs to distill our learning into the basic principles of psychodynamic psychopharmacology.

I also acknowledge the medical directors at Riggs under whom I served and learned, especially Eric Plakun, M.D., whose editorial eye sharpened my thinking and who supported me in bringing this project to completion.

I also acknowledge all of those who volunteered their time and minds to review and improve initial drafts of this work, in particular Patrick Kelly, who brought his writing skills and layman's eye to the task and helped me explain myself better; Elizabeth Weinberg, who brought her psychoanalyst's eye to the task and helped me see where I had not gone far enough; Louis Graff, M.D., and Madeleine Lansky, M.D., who brought the perspective of the clinician in the trenches and helped ensure these ideas were scalable; and Kate Gallagher, Ph.D., who did all of the above.

• PART I •

What Is Psychodynamic Psychopharmacology?

CHAPTER 1

What Is Psychodynamic Psychopharmacology?

We physicians cannot discard psychotherapy, if only because another person intimately concerned in the process of recovery—the patient—has no intention of discarding it....A factor dependent on the psychical disposition of the patient contributes, without any intention on our part, to the effect of every therapeutic process initiated by a physician; most frequently it is favorable to recovery, but often it acts as an inhibition....All physicians, therefore, yourselves included, are continually practicing psychotherapy, even when you have no intention of doing so and are not aware of it; it is a disadvantage, however, to leave the mental factor in your treatment so completely in the patient's hands. Thus it is impossible to keep a check on it, to administer it in doses or to intensify it. Is it not then a justifiable endeavor on the part of a physician to seek to obtain command of this factor, to use it with a purpose, and to direct and strengthen it?

—Sigmund Freud, *On Psychotherapy* (1905[1904]/1953)

Medications exert their effects via multiple pathways. Some are mediated biologically via their actions at various receptor sites, whereas others are mediated symbolically through the meanings they have for patients and the doctor–patient relationship (Mintz and Flynn 2012). The impact of psychosocial factors on medication outcomes is why the gold standard of evidence-based medicine is the placebo-controlled trial. The placebo effect, comprising a range of psychological and interpersonal factors, exerts a significant influence on the outcome of medical treatments, making it necessary to isolate this effect to determine the contribution of the medication to outcomes.

A burgeoning but still oft-neglected body of evidence suggests that nonpharmacological or nonspecific factors in pharmacotherapy are at least as potent as the putative "active ingredients" in a medication (Greenberg 2016;

Mintz and Flynn 2012; also see Chapter 3). For example, meta-analyses reviewing the FDA databases, which include a relatively unbiased sample of both published and unpublished data from antidepressant clinical trials, suggest that 75%–81% of drug response can be attributed to nonpharmacological effects, such as placebo (Khan et al. 2000; Kirsch and Sapirstein 1998; Kirsch et al. 2002). Other research from well-designed placebo-controlled trials shows that a strong pharmacotherapeutic alliance is an even more powerful antidepressant than the actual drugs prescribed (Krupnick et al. 1996). Similarly, an intriguing line of research suggests that, at least where antidepressants are concerned, prescribers contribute as much or even more to medication outcomes than the medication itself (McKay et al. 2006).

Despite considerable evidence that these meaning effects are central to medication response, there is no widely accepted method for incorporating this evidence base into clinical practice. Psychodynamic psychopharmacology (Mintz and Belnap 2006, 2011) emerged as an approach to optimizing treatment outcomes by integrating pharmacotherapy with evidence-based and psychodynamically informed perspectives that enhances therapeutic factors for the patient and in the doctor–patient encounter. It strengthens a traditional objective-descriptive, population-based approach with a patient-centered, psychodynamically informed awareness. Working together, these approaches pave the way for personalizing treatment. Factors such as meaning effects, therapeutic alliance, ambivalence, and patient autonomy have a powerful and measurable impact on the outcome of pharmacotherapy and must be considered if we are to treat the whole person. Psychodynamic psychopharmacology brings these elements together into a coherent model of treatment that is simultaneously personalized and evidence based.

Psychodynamic psychopharmacology explicitly recognizes that psychological and interpersonal factors play a crucial role in treatment outcome. It draws on extant frameworks for understanding the often-complex intersection of the patient's relationship to illness, caregivers, medications, and treatment. The literature provides important guidance for shaping the prescribing process and the doctor–patient relationship in order to optimize treatment outcomes. The extant evidence base focuses largely on "common factors" (Frank 1971), such as instilling hope and establishing a working alliance. These factors have robust effects that are now increasingly understood to apply to treatment outcomes not only in psychotherapy but also in psychopharmacotherapy (Bickman 2005; Davidson and Chan 2014) and medical care (Scovern 1999). Psychodynamic psychopharmacology, in seeing these factors through a psychodynamic lens, extends, deepens, and helps personalize them. In doing so, it recognizes that patients have multilayered wishes for treatment and that some of these desires may be in conflict and some may be unconscious. In this sense, psychodynamic psychopharmacology can be seen as providing a way to address antitherapeutic common factors likely to have adverse consequences on treatment outcome, such as patient ambivalence, experiences of disempowerment, and development of secondary gains (in which the rewards of illness may not even rise to the level of conscious awareness).

A common example is the patient who emphatically tells her new psychiatrist that she wants her depression to go away. Although this is undoubtedly true, the patient is generally unaware of the ways in which she *does not* want to lose her depression. From childhood she has believed that she always cared dutifully for others but almost never received any care in return. It is not hard to understand how she may feel covertly gratified by the care she now receives as a woman with depression and by the opportunity to be freed from the burden of caring for others while she convalesces. If she could lose the depression without losing the care she is receiving, she would. Unfortunately, given her past experience, she deeply experiences this as an either/or proposition, leaving her in a dilemma. That dilemma, however, is hardly conscious, because the patient has little or no awareness that she has become attached to her illness through the secondary gains it offers, but it is perhaps not surprising when she regularly forgets to take her antidepressant.

Psychodynamic psychopharmacology offers a framework for empathically appreciating that patients, and especially treatment-resistant patients, are likely in conflict around aspects of treatment. In this case, the barely registered conflict between being a caregiver and receiving care results in repeated nonadherence to treatment, which can adversely affect the outcome in myriad ways. Psychodynamic psychopharmacology also delivers a coherent model that integrates unique aspects of patients' psychology with the evidence bases that connect meaning and medications. This model provides doctors with recommendations and tools for helping patients become aware of their ambivalences about and resistances to treatment so that these can be addressed directly within the unfolding doctor–patient alliance, removing impediments to a good outcome and helping to restore patients to a healthier relationship with illness, treatment, and caregiving.

The unfortunate and unintended consequences of psychiatry's biomedical emphasis and narrow focus on the evidence base are becoming clearer. One is that the doctor, who is presumed to have mastery of the evidence base, is positioned as the expert. This dynamic puts the doctor more in charge and places the patient in a subordinate position. At the same time, the focus on medications as the primary curative agent locates all of the healing power in the doctor and the doctor's medications. There are probably some good reasons for emphasizing the potency of medications; evidence has shown that high expectations of medications, in both the patient (Aikens et al. 2005: Gaudiano and Miller 2006; Krell et al. 2004; Meyer et al. 2002) and the doctor (Uhlenhuth et al. 1966), can contribute to a robust treatment response. However, taken together, these developments in the culture of mental health have the subtle effect of deauthorizing patients and putting them in a passive role in their mental health treatment.

By recognizing that patients' attitudes, fears, and wishes are major determinants of treatment outcome, psychodynamic psychopharmacology helps restore balance when treatment approaches have overly reduced treatment resistance to a problem of biology. Restoring a measure of responsibility for treatment outcome to patients empowers them to move out of the passive role of waiting to be cured by the doctor and into a more active role in their recovery process. To this end, psychodynamic prescribers support patient agency by educating patients about the impact of psychosocial factors on treatment outcomes, working with them to illuminate their fears and deeper wishes in relation to treatment, and allowing what is learned through this process to guide the prescribing process.

The theory and techniques of psychodynamic psychopharmacology developed out of work with patients who presented with psychopharmacological treatment resistance. However, given the universality of common factors and the complex feelings patients have about illness and treatment, such techniques likely would also benefit psychiatry patients without demonstrated treatment resistance. It may well be that applying a patient-centered, psychodynamically informed approach to prescribing decreases the emergence of chronification (Isler 1988) and treatment resistance. The recommendations offered in this book are also likely generalizable to patients with chronic medical conditions who rely on medications to manage their illness.

Furthermore, psychodynamic psychopharmacology recognizes that many of the foundational insights of psychoanalysis (e.g., the unconscious, conflict, resistance, transference, defense) are powerful factors in the complex relationships between the patient, the illness, the doctor, and the medication. As Freud (1905[1904]/1953) noted, these factors are often concordant with therapeutic aims (i.e., placebo effect), in which case they naturally support positive outcomes. In other cases, however, patients grapple with conscious and unconscious factors that conflict with important aspects of treatment, worsening outcomes. The presence of psychological and social factors that conflict with treatment or its aims should therefore be considered when patients present with highly treatment-resistant or unexpectedly chronic conditions.

When patients' treatment resistance derives from the level of meaning, it will most effectively be addressed at that same level. Strictly biomedical interventions, such as changing medications or dosages, will likely encounter the same sources of resistance that previously interfered with a therapeutic response. Prescribers who are working within a primarily biomedical framework likely will not have the tools necessary to address the psychological and interpersonal sources of treatment resistance. Psychodynamic psychopharmacology is grounded in the understanding that outcomes can be improved when doctors understand the different meanings that illness and treatment have for their patients. Such an understanding allows them to focus on patients' varied and often conflicting goals to support healthy strivings, explicitly address ambivalence, make resistances available for exploration, and confront covertly countertherapeutic uses of treatment.

The doctor–patient relationship is an important vehicle of change that can either interfere with or support patients' healthy use of medications. Psychodynamic pharmacology draws on both an emerging evidence base that points to the effects of alliance on pharmacotherapy outcomes and an understanding of the role of transference as both a resistance to treatment and a vehicle of growth. This enhances clinicians' ability to form a working alliance that is in tune with their patients' goals (as conflicting as those goals may be) and empowers patients to take a more active role in recovery.

When the meanings of treatment and illness, patients' overall aims in life, the doctor–patient relationship, and patients' authority are explicitly engaged in the prescribing process, patients, rather than illness, become the center of treatment. A dehumanizing, reductionistic symptom focus is countered when symptoms are addressed not as problems in their own right but specifically in terms of how they interfere with patients' functioning and broader life goals. Recognizing that patients' goals may be in conflict allows patients and their doctors to grapple with some basic conflicts of life as they pertain to psychiatric care. For example, when a patient who wishes not to feel depressed also benefits from a caring attentiveness that he or she would not otherwise receive, it is useful to make such conflicts explicit so that the patient and doctor can focus on them. Otherwise, this conflict operates in the shadows, and the patient will have little control over such unconscious influences.

The traditional medical model of treatment positions the doctor as the expert. In many ways, this has only become more entrenched as the evidence base has been reified, positioning doctors as masters of the evidence base. Because this evidence base is focused largely on medications, particularly in psychiatry, patients are often at risk of becoming disempowered as they wait for the doctor's treatments to work. Psychodynamic psychopharmacology offers an antidote to this potential danger. By emphasizing evidence bases that suggest patients' psychology and involvement in treatment are crucial, it reinvests part of the authority for treatment outcomes back in the patient while still being guided by the evidence, leading to better outcomes.

Key Points

- Psychodynamic psychopharmacology integrates psychodynamic insights with patient-centered and evidence-based approaches to prescribing.

- Psychodynamic psychopharmacology explicitly recognizes that psychological and interpersonal factors play a crucial role in treatment outcome.

- Psychodynamic psychopharmacology offers a framework for empathically appreciating that patients, especially those resistant to treatment, are likely in conflict around aspects of that treatment.

- Psychodynamic psychopharmacology recognizes that, in pharmacotherapy, the prescriber–patient relationship is an important vehicle for change.

- Focusing on psychological and interpersonal factors in pharmacotherapy promotes patients' agency as an active factor in recovery using pharmacotherapy.

References

Aikens JE, Kroenke K, Swindle RW, et al: Nine-month predictors and outcomes of SSRI antidepressant continuation in primary care. Gen Hosp Psychiatry 27(4):229–236, 2005 15993253

Bickman L: A common factors approach to improving mental health services. Ment Health Serv Res 7(1):1–4, 2005 15832689

Davidson L, Chan KK: Common factors: evidence-based practice and recovery. Psychiatr Serv 65(5):675–677, 2014 24535634

Frank JD: Eleventh Emil A. Gutheil memorial conference: therapeutic factors in psychotherapy. Am J Psychother 25(3):350–361, 1971 4936109

Freud S: On psychotherapy (1905[1904]), in Standard Edition of the Complete Psychological Works of Sigmund Freud, Vol 7. Translated and edited by Strachey J. London, Hogarth, 1953, pp 257–270

Gaudiano BA, Miller IW: Patients' expectancies, the alliance in pharmacotherapy, and treatment outcomes in bipolar disorder. J Consult Clin Psychol 74(4):671–676, 2006

Greenberg RP: The rebirth of psychosocial importance in a drug-filled world. Am Psychol 71(8):781–791, 2016 27977264

Isler H: Headache drugs provoking chronic headache: historical aspects and common misunderstandings, in Drug-Induced Headache. (Advances in Applied Neurological Sciences, Vol 5. Edited by Diener HC, Wilkinson M). New York, Springer, 1988, pp 87–94

Khan A, Warner HA, Brown WA: Symptom reduction and suicide risk in patients treated with placebo in antidepressant clinical trials: an analysis of the Food and Drug Administration database. Arch Gen Psychiatry 57(4):311–317, 2000 10768687

Kirsch I, Sapirstein G: Listening to Prozac but hearing placebo: a meta-analysis of antidepressant medication. Prevention and Treatment 1(2), 1998

Kirsch I, Moore TJ, Scoboria A, et al: The emperor's new drugs: an analysis of antidepressant medication data submitted to the U.S. Food and Drug Administration. Prevention and Treatment 5(23), 2002

Krell HV, Leuchter AF, Morgan M, et al: Subject expectations of treatment effectiveness and outcome of treatment with an experimental antidepressant. J Clin Psychiatry 65(9):1174–1179, 2004 15367043

Krupnick JL, Sotsky SM, Simmens S, et al: The role of the therapeutic alliance in psychotherapy and pharmacotherapy outcome: findings in the National Institute of Mental Health Treatment of Depression Collaborative Research Program. J Consult Clin Psychol 64(3):532–539, 1996 8698947

McKay KM, Imel ZE, Wampold BE: Psychiatrist effects in the psychopharmacological treatment of depression. J Affect Disord 92(2–3):287–290, 2006 16503356

Meyer B, Pilkonis PA, Krupnick JL, et al: Treatment expectancies, patient alliance, and outcome: further analyses from the National Institute of Mental Health Treatment of Depression Collaborative Research Program. J Consult Clin Psychol 70(4):1051–1055, 2002 12182269

Mintz D, Belnap B: A view from Riggs—treatment resistance and patient authority, III: what is psychodynamic psychopharmacology? An approach to pharmacologic treatment resistance. J Am Acad Psychoanal Dyn Psychiatry 34(4):581–601, 2006 17274730

Mintz DL, Belnap B: What is psychodynamic psychopharmacology? An approach to pharmacological treatment resistance, in Treatment Resistance and Patient Authority: The Austen Riggs Reader. Edited by Plakun E. New York, WW Norton, 2011, pp 42–65

Mintz DL, Flynn DF: How (not what) to prescribe: nonpharmacologic aspects of psychopharmacology. Psychiatr Clin North Am 35(1):143–163, 2012 22370496

Scovern AW: From placebo to alliance: the role of common factors in medicine, in The Heart and Soul of Change: What Works in Therapy. Edited by Hubble MA, Duncan BL, Miller SD. Washington, DC, American Psychological Association, 1999, pp 259–295

Uhlenhuth EH, Rickels K, Fisher S, et al: Drug, doctor's verbal attitude and clinic setting in the symptomatic response to pharmacotherapy. Psychopharmacology (Berl) 9(5):392–418, 1966 4872909

• CHAPTER 2 •

Why Psychodynamic Psychopharmacology?

If anyone thinks he can exclude philosophy and leave it aside as useless he will be eventually defeated by it in some obscure form or other.

—Karl Jaspers, *General Psychopathology* (1913)

As detailed in Chapter 1, psychodynamic psychopharmacology integrates biomedical psychiatry with psychodynamic insights and techniques. This effort to bridge biomedical and psychodynamic psychiatry and to incorporate evidence bases about psychosocial aspects of medication into the prescribing process was undertaken in response to the growing recognition of treatment resistance in psychiatry. Although debates over the relative importance of the *science* of medicine (what to do) versus the *art* of medicine (how to do it) are as old as modern medicine itself, the growth of medical science and technologies since the second half of the 20th century has tended to favor science at the expense of an integrated, person-centered perspective. Various attempts have been made to move the field of medicine back toward integration, including Balint's ideas of "the overall diagnosis" and "patient-centered medicine" (Balint and Norell 2001) and the "biopsychosocial model" proposed by Engel (1977). Despite acceptance of these ideas, their impact on clinical practice has been curtailed by real-world pressures, lack of a coherent model of care delivery, and lack of resources to develop an evidence base.

For much of the 20th century, the psychoanalytic model was in ascendance. Psychological reductionism was the greater risk to integration, with patients held responsible in some form for their emotional distress and a range of medical pathologies that were identified as psychosomatic. Although Freud saw himself as working within a medical model, pharmacotherapy was often viewed as an inferior mode of treatment, creating a polarization in the field of mental health. As effective medications were discovered and created,

11

many of the key insights of the psychodynamic era were discarded, and psychological reductionism gave way to biomedical reductionism. This polarization was exacerbated by the pharmaceutical industry, which contributed to the medicalization of human suffering, and then by the increasing influence of managed care, in which concerns about efficiency and cost-effectiveness often trump concerns related to clinical effectiveness. These pressures outside of psychiatry joined with the excitement within psychiatry about our burgeoning understanding in the neurosciences. As mentioned in the preface to this book, the National Institute of Mental Health (NIMH) began channeling its resources into research with demonstrable biomedical targets and essentially stopped funding research into psychosocial aspects of care.

A reductionistic approach, however, is bound to be limited by what is excluded. Psychiatry, under this biomedical model, fell under the sway of several false or overly limiting assumptions (Plakun 2018), including the ideas that genes equal disease, that patients present with single disorders that respond to specific evidence-based treatments, and that the best treatments are pills. Treatment algorithms addressing treatment-refractory psychiatric conditions typically advocated diagnostic clarity and more or different medications, with little recognition of or guidance about psychosocial aspects of care that might ameliorate treatment resistance. In this algorithm, for example (Figure 2–1), which is unusual in its effort to recognize that clinical and psychosocial complexity might contribute to treatment resistance, there is no guidance about how to address such complexity except to "manage accordingly."

Ultimately, the limitations of this model became increasingly apparent. Thomas Insel, who directed the NIMH and oversaw the adoption of the Research Domain Criteria, concluded at the end of his tenure:

> I spent 13 years at NIMH really pushing on the neuroscience and genetics of mental disorders, and when I look back on that I realize that while I think I succeeded at getting lots of really cool papers published by cool scientists at fairly large costs—I think $20 billion—I don't think we moved the needle in reducing suicide, reducing hospitalizations, improving recovery for the tens of millions of people who have mental illness. (Rogers 2017)

Psychodynamic psychopharmacology attempts to understand what it means to "manage accordingly" when clinical and psychosocial complexity interfere with optimal response to psychopharmacotherapy. It also answers the greater call toward a more patient-centered approach (Epstein et al. 2010) focused not only on symptoms but also on function (Rush and Thase 2018) and recognizes that pills are not, in themselves, the answer. Rather, this approach understands that what is needed is a method that also empowers patients by incorporating a long-term focus on behavioral and attitude change

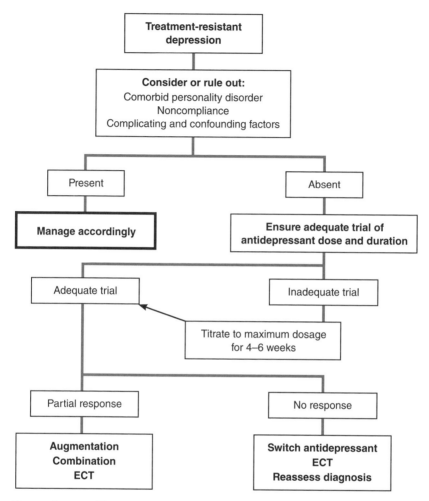

Figure 2–1. Treatment algorithm for treatment-resistant depression.

ECT = electroconvulsive therapy.
Source. Adapted from Chehil et al. 2001.

(Rush and Thase 2018) into a traditional medical approach. This chapter reviews some of the evidence base regarding both the problem of treatment resistance and what is known about the contribution of psychosocial factors to treatment resistance and pharmacological outcomes, underlining the reasons that call for a psychodynamic response. Other potential benefits of psychodynamic psychopharmacology are also explored.

The Problem of Treatment Resistance

Psychodynamic psychopharmacology developed in response to the significant problem of pharmacological treatment resistance. Unfortunately, there is little evidence that advances in neuroscientific understanding or drug development have fostered substantially better outcomes for patients with psychiatric illness. Quite to the contrary, in the psychiatric literature since the 1980s, there has been a 7,500% increase in references to treatment-resistant psychiatric conditions. In the 5-year period from 1980 through 1984, there were 36 references to treatment-resistant psychiatric conditions. That number has increased exponentially every 5 years, so that between 2010 and 2014, there were 2,696 references in the medical literature to treatment-resistant psychiatric conditions (Figure 2–2). To some extent, this reflects improvements in our ability to understand and use the evidence base so that we are more aware of the limitations of current psychiatric practice. However, evidence suggests that the actual problem of depression and treatment-resistant depression is growing, not shrinking (Kessler et al. 2003).

At least 15% and as many as 50% of psychiatric patients will to respond adequately to pharmacotherapy (Berlim and Turecki 2007; Lieberman et al. 2005; Perlis et al. 2006; Thase et al. 2001, 2007). Evidence from trials such as the Sequenced Treatment Alternatives to Relieve Depression (STAR*D; Thase et al. 2007) suggests that even with multiple medications, including augmentation strategies, treatment resistance remains a significant issue. Even when patients have a clinically meaningful response to medications, most seem to be left with such significant residual symptoms that any reasonable person with those symptoms would seek treatment (Westen and Morrison 2001). The problem of treatment resistance only becomes more significant when we consider not only "ideal patients" with single disorders but also outcomes with real-world patients with complex, comorbid psychiatric conditions, including personality pathology (Bender et al. 2006; Plakun 2018; Skodol et al. 2005, 2011). These findings point not only to the limitations of our current medications but also to challenges that exist in the patients' psychology, the prescribing process, or the doctor–patient relationship. Evidence suggests that roughly one-third of patients are completely noncompliant with their prescribed medications (Cramer and Rosenheck 1998), and another third are only partially compliant (Boudes 1998). For example, in the Clinical Antipsychotic Trials in Intervention Effectiveness (CATIE; Lieberman et al. 2005) study, only about one-quarter of patients with schizophrenia remained adherent to psychopharmacotherapy after 18 months of treatment.

How are we to understand the problem of increasing treatment resistance in an era of optimism about our growing understanding of the neurobiology of mental illness? As biologically reductionistic approaches dominate

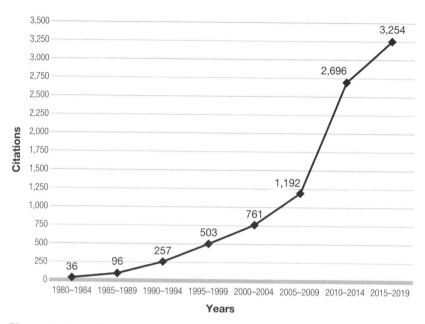

Figure 2–2.   Treatment resistance in the psychiatric literature.

psychiatric practice, patient care has steered away from considering the potent effects of meaning and relationships in psychopharmacological treatment. By construing patients as passive recipients of concrete, specific, and straightforward medical interventions, the field has succumbed to a "delusion of precision" (Gutheil 1982) and unwittingly moved into an era of treatment resistance in which some of our most potent tools are wasted. Such a reductionistic focus may not only deprive treaters of flexibility in adapting to the complex problems of people with psychiatric symptoms but also contribute directly to treatment resistance. As Plakun (2006) noted, for some patients, resisting treatments may be their best effort to counter a medical system that they experience as reducing them from a person to an illness. These patients may attempt to reestablish a sense of equilibrium and control by refusing to follow the psychopharmacologist's treatment recommendations, taking either too little or too much medication according to their own wishes, or refusing treatment altogether.

Psychodynamic psychopharmacology enhances traditional approaches that consider adequacy of dosage, duration of treatment, and correctness of diagnosis. To these approaches it adds an understanding of potential psychodynamics operating in the patient and the doctor–patient dyad that may promote treatment resistance.

The Meaning of Medication

Pills are not just psychoactive substances held together with binding agents. Rather, pills are powerfully symbolic, carrying a broad range of personal and interpersonal meanings that can have wide-ranging effects on a patient's psychology, neurobiology (Mayberg et al. 2002), and functioning. The psychosocial dimension of psychopharmacology consists of multiple factors that expert prescribers would do well to understand, ranging from the actual physical characteristics of pills, to the psychosocial characteristics of patients and prescribers, to the quality of the doctor–patient relationship. In fact, in much of the research on medication outcome, psychosocial factors appear to be more potent than the putative active ingredients of the medications, at least as far as antidepressants are concerned (Ankarberg and Falkenström 2008). A series of meta-analyses reviewing antidepressant effectiveness in the FDA database (a sample untainted by publication bias) suggested, for example, that 75%–81% of drug response can be attributed to the placebo response (Khan et al. 2000; Kirsch and Sapirstein 1998; Kirsch et al. 2002). Not only are these changes clinically meaningful, but further evidence also suggests that, in many cases, placebo benefits are also persisting (Khan et al. 2008). Psychodynamic psychopharmacology, as an approach to treatment resistance, recognizes that the best evidence supports a major role for psychosocial aspects of medications and attempts to capitalize on this factor to optimize outcomes.

Physical Characteristics of the Pill

Factors as prosaic as the color of the pill (de Craen et al. 1996; Fisher and Greenberg 1997) appear to significantly influence the actions of medications. In Western nations, red pills are superior at generating energizing effects, whereas blue pills, in general, are more calming, reducing both anxiety (Schapira et al. 1970) and depression (de Craen et al. 1996). Curiously, however, this effect is reversed in Italian men (Cattaneo et al. 1970), for whom the color blue does not reflect the metaphor of tranquility but rather is connected to images of vitality and energy; this culture-specific placebo effect is thought to be connected to the Italian soccer team "The Blues." Other clinically meaningful characteristics of a medication include its expense, because there appears to be a direct correlation between the perceived expense of a pill and its effectiveness (Waber et al. 2008), and its route of administration, in which more intrusive administrations (e.g., parenteral) are more potent (de Craen et al. 2000; Kaptchuk et al. 2000).

The finding that the characteristics of a pill affect treatment response is not just a curiosity. Given the ubiquity of generic substitutions, changes in the nonpharmacological characteristics of medications are a reality that patients regularly encounter and can have demonstrated effects on treatment outcome. For example, patients receiving generic substitutions report a decreased intention to continue taking the medication (Roman 2009). Furthermore, up to 34% of patients with new generic substitutes experience adverse medication effects that cannot be explained by pharmacological activity (Weissenfeld et al. 2010). Integrating an understanding of the adverse effects of generic substitutions (in which patients often feel powerless) into the prescribing process may counter some of the negative effects.

Psychosocial Characteristics of Patients That Affect Treatment Outcomes

A broad range of factors affects the actions of medications, many of which relate to the maturity of patients' psychological functioning or to patients' sense of autonomy and self-efficacy (Table 2–1). Psychodynamic psychopharmacologists are in the best position to optimize those psychosocial factors in patients that will promote good outcomes. Similarly, they are better attuned to and able to address those factors in patients that can interfere with pharmacological treatment. Less mature defenses (e.g., denial, splitting, projective identification) appear, for example, to be a poor prognostic sign for pharmacotherapy in patients with depression (Kronström et al. 2009). Similarly, there is an inverse correlation between the degree of neuroticism (relative immaturity of defenses together with a tendency toward worry and dysphoria) and short- and long-term medication response (Joyce and Paykel 1989; Scott et al. 1995), at least regarding antidepressant response. These patients also have a higher risk of depressive recurrence (Steunenberg et al. 2010), and medications alone are especially unlikely to be adequate treatment (Ghaemi et al. 2012).

Attachment styles (Bartholomew and Horowitz 1991), defined as fundamental modes of relating to others that are partly shaped by early caregiving relationships, also significantly affect the ways medications are used. People with secure attachments are able comfortably to connect to and separate from important others and have a basic sense of trust. Anxious-fearful attachment patterns, similar to those with sociotropy, are characterized by feelings of interpersonal insecurity and worries about evoking a negative response from important others. People with dismissive or avoidant attachments readily disconnect from others at the first disappointment; these are the "one strike and you're out" patients who often show particular difficulty with treatment adherence (Ciechanowski et al. 2001). Patients with secure attachments show an earlier response to antidepressants than patients with fearful attachments (Comninos and Grenyer 2007). An understanding of the

Table 2–1.   Nonpharmacological pharmacotherapy variables affecting
              outcomes

Psychosocial variable	Supporting studies
Acquiescence	Fast and Fisher 1971; McNair et al. 1968, 1970
Ambivalence about medications	Aikens et al. 2008; Sirey et al. 2001; Warden et al. 2009
Attachment style	Ciechanowski et al. 2001, 2006; Comninos and Grenyer 2007
Autonomous motivation for treatment	Zuroff et al. 2007
Autonomy	Peselow et al. 1992
Defensive style	Kronström et al. 2009
Early trauma	Williams et al. 2016
Expectations of treatment	Aikens et al. 2005; Gaudiano and Miller 2006; Krell et al. 2004; Meyer et al. 2002; Sneed et al. 2008
Locus of control	Reynaert et al. 1995
Neuroticism	Bagby et al. 2002; Joyce and Paykel 1989; Scott et al. 1995; Steunenberg et al. 2010
Readiness to change	Beitman et al. 1994; Lewis et al. 2009
Secondary gains associated with illness	van Egmond and Kummeling 2002
Social disadvantage	Hahn 1997
Sociotropy	Peselow et al. 1992
Theory of illness	Sullivan et al. 2003
Treatment preference	Iacoviello et al. 2007; Kocsis et al. 2009; Kwan et al. 2010; Lin et al. 2005; Raue et al. 2009

patient's attachment style may offer the prescribing clinician guidance about how to prescribe because evidence suggests that nonadherence associated with dismissive attachments can be ameliorated by particularly good communication on the part of the doctor (Ciechanowski et al. 2001). These patients may also respond better to a team-based collaborative care approach (Ciechanowski et al. 2006) that offers extended support.

Locus of control (Rotter 1966), the extent to which individuals believe that the outcomes of their behavior are a function of internal factors (e.g., own behavior, personal characteristics), exerts significant effects on medication response. Patients with an internal locus of control fare significantly better with antidepressants than those whose external locus of control leads them to believe that external factors (e.g., other people's behavior, situational characteristics) determine their outcomes (Reynaert et al. 1995). Similarly, autonomy (a sense of independence and self-efficacy) and sociotropy are personality characteristics that impact pharmacological treatment outcome, the former directly and the latter inversely (Peselow et al. 1992). Patients exhibiting high autonomy and low sociotropy have an increased likelihood of a positive antidepressant response rate (74.1%) compared with those with high sociotropy and low autonomy (38.5%).

Patients with sociotropy may paradoxically impair themselves in the context of pharmacological treatment, handing too much responsibility for cure over to the doctor and emptying themselves of personal efficacy. One intriguing line of research comparing outcomes of psychotherapy alone versus psychotherapy plus a placebo pill supports this hypothesis. Hollon and DeRubeis (1981) pointed to the fact that patients receiving the combination had worse outcomes than the patients receiving only psychotherapy. They suggested that these patients had worse outcomes because they were less motivated to work hard in therapy and were waiting for the pill to work instead. Furthermore, research on the role of self-efficacy on pharmacological treatment found that patients who view their depression as primarily "psychological" benefit more from antidepressant treatment (Sullivan et al. 2003) than those who see their depression as "biological."

Feelings of disempowerment may not only reduce the benefits of medications but also increase the potential for harm. The *nocebo effect* (Kennedy 1961), the converse of the placebo response, occurs when patients who harbor expectations of harm are more likely to respond adversely to medications (Mintz 2002). An experience of powerlessness seems to be particularly fertile ground for nocebo responses. Individuals from socially disadvantaged groups (e.g., minorities, women, those of low socioeconomic status) are more nocebo prone (Hahn 1997), as are people who characteristically acquiesce to the wishes of others (Fast and Fisher 1971; McNair et al. 1968, 1970). These patients can become treatment resistant when medication trials are repeatedly interrupted by intolerable side effects or when therapeutic dosages are never achieved because of the patient's sensitivity to side effects. Importantly, the nocebo effect can occur regardless of whether the expectation of harm is conscious or unconscious (Jensen et al. 2012). Personality styles also play a role in proneness to side effects. Patients with neuroticism, for example, tend to be more prone to side effect reporting (Davis et al. 1995). Although the reasons for treatment resistance in this population are complicated, one potential source is that adequate dosages and durations of treatment could not be attained because of the patients' proneness to the nocebo effect.

At the same time, there is evidence that a disempowering relationship to medications can worsen outcomes. In fact, studies suggest that patients with higher expectations of pharmacological treatment experience more immediate benefit. For instance, patients receiving active drugs in studies in which they know they will receive an antidepressant show antidepressant response rates of approximately 60%. However, when patients are told that they may receive a placebo, their response to the active drug drops to 46% (Sneed et al. 2008). Indeed, whereas patients with high expectations of medications had an impressive 90% antidepressant response rate, patients who had only moderate expectations of treatment responded only 33% of the time (Krell et al. 2004). Several other studies (e.g., Rutherford et al. 2010) have supported the idea that expectancies play a major role in medication outcome, although this effect may be moderated partly by effects on the therapeutic alliance in the treatment of patients with major depression (Meyer et al. 2002) or bipolar disorder (Gaudiano and Miller 2006).

Although patients most often present for treatment voluntarily, in the hope of being relieved of their psychiatric distress, they also are often deeply ambivalent about pharmacological treatment. In some cases, this ambivalence stems from worries about being harmed by medications, worries that appear to be quite common. In a study of patients' mental representations of antidepressant medications, themes of harm outweighed themes of clinical benefit. Of 17 themes to emerge from patients' narratives about antidepressant treatment, causing adverse effects (56%) and creating dependency (47%) were the two most prevalent themes, followed by soothing (44%) and improving mood (39%) (Piguet et al. 2007). Particularly with psychiatric medications, harm may not only be experienced as physical harm but also be particularly infused with threats to identity and stigmatizing social meanings (Pound et al. 2005). Patients' ambivalence about treatment has profound clinical implications. Ambivalence about medications is a major contributor to treatment nonadherence. Aikens et al. (2005) found that initial skepticism about the appropriateness of pharmacological treatment resulted in significant increases in antidepressant discontinuation. Moreover, patients who express early ambivalence are also twice as likely to discontinue medications prematurely and three times more likely to stop medications prematurely in the context of side effects (Warden et al. 2009). Perceived stigma about taking psychiatric medications is also known to predict antidepressant nonadherence (Sirey et al. 2001).

Patients also are often ambivalent about their illness itself. Studies suggest that approximately one-half of patients can identify secondary benefits of illness (Dulgar-Tulloch 2009; van Egmond et al. 2005). Secondary gain from illness renders them much less likely to experience remission of symptoms (van Egmond and Kummeling 2002). Although patients may not become ill because of the secondary gains of their illness, it is understandable and even healthy to try, consciously or unconsciously, to secure some benefit from a bad situation. In this way, however, patients may become quite at-

Table 2–2.   Characteristics of the prescriber that may affect outcome

Agreement about targets	Nonauthoritarian communication style
Attitudes toward drug therapy	Respect for treatment preferences
Empathy	Positive affectivity or voice tone
Focus on the patient (as opposed to a digital display)	Psychological theory of illness
	Shared decision making
Good communication	Warmth
Investment in the patient and symptomatic improvement	

tached to their symptoms. Symptoms and illness behaviors may come to represent their best efforts at managing overwhelming affect, communicating something that cannot be put into words, or eluding intolerable living situations (Mintz and Belnap 2006, 2011).

Similarly, patients' "readiness to change" seems to be another factor that is more important for pharmacological treatment response than treatment with an active drug. Beitman et al. (1994) found that among patients treated for anxiety, those who received a benzodiazepine and were highly motivated to change had the most robust response. However, patients receiving placebo who were highly motivated to change had a greater reduction in anxiety than precontemplative (less motivated) patients who received the active drug. Readiness to change was found to be the single most powerful determinant of treatment effectiveness, even more potent than drug condition (i.e., active vs. placebo). This finding has been replicated for patients with depressive disorders as well (Lewis et al. 2009).

Prescriber Characteristics

Who the prescriber is and how he or she prescribes may exert as much of an effect on treatment outcomes as what is prescribed, particularly in relation to antidepressants (Table 2–2). A robust example of this comes from a secondary analysis of data from the Treatment of Depression Collaborative Research Program (TDCRP), an extensive NIMH-funded, multicenter, placebo-controlled trial of the treatment of depression (McKay et al. 2006). In this study, McKay et al. (2006) sought to compare the relative effects of the prescriber versus the drug condition (i.e., active or placebo). They found large differences in treatment outcomes between different prescribers, even though experimental conditions tightly controlled most aspects of the doctor–patient engagement. Using linear hierarchical modeling, they stratified outcomes by prescriber: one-third of the psychiatrists in the study could be described as highly effective, achieving superior results with active drug and placebo; another third exhibited average performance, and another third were relatively ineffective. More striking, perhaps, is the fact that the most effective group of prescribers achieved better outcomes with placebos than the least effective group of prescribers achieved with active antidepressants.

What did the more effective prescribers do in the TDCRP study? It was already well known that prescribers who present as warm (Rickels et al. 1971) or empathetic (Downing et al. 1973) tend to elicit more robust therapeutic effects from prescribed medications. Analysis of clinician effects (including both prescribers and psychotherapists) in this study supported these earlier findings (Blatt et al. 1996a, 1996b). The more caring, empathic, open, and sincere that patients experienced their doctors to be, the better their outcome ratings became. The more effective prescribers also had in common a psychological rather than biological orientation to treating depression and appeared to place less unitary emphasis on medication. Although there are likely many ways that a psychological perspective on patients benefits pharmacological treatments, one likely mechanism is that this way of working is experienced by patients as empathic. Indeed, a psychodynamic formulation of their patients' troubles is known to help treaters preserve a measure of empathy in working with even the most challenging patients (Treloar 2009). Empathy, in turn, is well known to support positive outcomes across a range of treatments and medical conditions (e.g., Kaplan et al. 2013; Squier 1990).

A biological theory of illness can have adverse consequences in psychiatric treatment (Sullivan et al. 2003). Such adverse effects can inadvertently be promoted by psychiatric caregivers when they espouse a biogenic theory of illness. For example, in one study of the effects of biogenic explanations, college students with a history of depression were ostensibly enrolled in a study to determine, by genetic testing, whether their depression was psychogenic or biogenic in origin. Subjects were randomized into biogenic or psychogenic groups. After a white-coated experimenter took a cheek swab "for analysis," the experimenter returned and told students the cause of their depression. Students who were informed that their depression was biological reported more prognostic pessimism and worsening mood-regulation expectancies (Kemp et al. 2014). Both prognostic pessimism (Rutherford et al. 2010) and mood-regulation expectancies (Kirsch et al. 1990) are known to affect outcome in depression. Other researchers (Deacon and Baird 2009; Lebowitz et al. 2013) have found similar effects of biogenic explanations in promoting attitudes that may undermine treatment outcomes. This does not mean, however, that prescribers should be dismissive toward medications, because this can adversely affect outcome as well. Therapeutic optimism promotes better outcomes, and prescribers can be trained to present themselves in such a manner (Uhlenhuth et al. 1966). Skilled prescribing involves not only conveying realistic optimism about the potential benefits of psychiatric treatment but also conveying realistic humility and finding hope in empowering patients to become active participants in the task of recovery.

Quality of the Doctor–Patient Relationship

The doctor–patient alliance seems to be at least as important for pharmacological treatment outcome as medication. An analysis of the TDCRP study examined the role of alliance in treatment outcomes in patients with depression (Krupnick et al. 1996). Patients had the best outcomes when a strong alliance was paired with the active drug. Furthermore, when they compared treatment conditions, researchers found that the patients receiving placebo who believed they had a good treatment alliance fared better than those who received the active antidepressant but had a poor alliance.

As noted, one aspect of a good therapeutic alliance hinges on the characteristics of the prescriber, including warmth and empathy. Warmth, as a variable, can be expressed in various ways. A warm tone of voice, for example, has been shown to have a substantial impact on whether patients show up for scheduled appointments: for every standard deviation interval above the mean of warmth in voice tone, there was a corresponding 162% increase in appointment adherence (Cruz et al. 2013). The presence of the prescriber emotionally, and even physically, also plays a major role in promoting an effective alliance. The prescriber's investment in the patient and in a positive outcome is correlated with positive outcomes (Lyerly et al. 1964). More frequent contact with doctors contributes to a strong alliance and is a factor in improved antidepressant adherence (Bull et al. 2002). The positive effects of frequent contact may be further amplified when it is paired with a supportive environment and involvement with family members (Frank et al. 1995).

Remaining present with patients is an increasing challenge in the era of the electronic medical record, in which pressures for efficiency and technology-driven interviews may mediate the doctor–patient relationship. Unfortunately, evidence indicates that when such technology draws the attention of the clinician, treatment suffers. One recent naturalistic study of treatment continuation found that when the doctor did not interact with the computer during an intake assessment for a psychiatric clinic, 77% of patients returned for a second appointment. If, however, the doctor interacted with a computer even once, only 27% of patients returned for a follow-up visit (Rosen et al. 2016). More important, a strong alliance also engages patients (or the healthier aspects of patients) in a spirit of shared inquiry and partnership and empowers them to become active participants in the healthy use of medications, which encourages long-term adherence (Frank et al. 1995). A stance that supports patients' autonomy also allows them to find their own autonomous motivation for treatment and appears to contribute substantially and positively to treatment outcomes (Zuroff et al. 2007).

One simple and important strategy for enhancing engagement is to elicit patients' preferences for type of treatment. Within the bounds of reason and conscience, it is useful to give patients the treatment they want, particularly if they hold strong preferences for one form of treatment over another (Raue et al. 2009). If a patient prefers medications to psychotherapy, the patient should be offered medications. The converse is even more true: patients who prefer psychotherapy should be offered psychotherapy because they are unlikely to benefit from medications. Kocsis et al. (2009) found that patients receiving their preferred treatments remitted approximately 45%–50% of the time. However, when receiving nonpreferred treatments, patients receiving psychotherapy showed a 22.2% remission rate, but those receiving medications remitted only 7.7% of the time! Patients who receive their preferred treatments appear also to benefit more rapidly than patients receiving nonpreferred treatments (Lin et al. 2005). It may be that treatment preferences exert their effects on outcome indirectly, via effects on other variables such as adherence and alliance. Patients assigned to nonpreferred treatments are less likely to even start treatment and are more likely to drop out after starting (Raue et al. 2009), particularly when treatment preferences are strong. Patients receiving nonpreferred treatments also attend fewer scheduled appointments with their doctors, accounting for as much as 16% of outcome variance (Kwan et al. 2010), but those receiving medications who prefer psychotherapy show significant decreases in alliance over the course of treatment (Iacoviello et al. 2007).

Beyond the type of treatment (e.g., medications vs. psychotherapy), there are other ways to involve patients in decision making, including selection of treatment goals, medication, and dosing schedule. Involving patients in this way enhances the alliance and increases their satisfaction with treatment (Loh et al. 2007). Perhaps more important, involving them in treatment decisions enhances their utilization of treatment. In one study (Woolley et al. 2010), inpatients and outpatients with depression who were involved in treatment decisions were 2.3 times more likely to continue taking their medications. Such involvement may be as simple as having a choice in the dosing schedule (e.g., once daily vs. three times daily). These patients were also twice as likely to discontinue treatment when they did not agree with the doctor's diagnosis. When patients disagreed with the diagnosis and felt uninvolved in decision making, they were 7.3 times more likely to discontinue treatment against recommendations. Patients involved in medical decision making have substantially better 18-month treatment outcomes (Clever et al. 2006), with the degree of involvement directly correlated with the degree of improvement. Involving patients in decision making also benefits treatments in more subtle ways, promoting treatment regimens that are ultimately more guideline concordant (Clever et al. 2006). Although busy prescribers might protest that they have insufficient time to elicit patients' preferences and to involve the patients in clinical decision making, available evidence suggests that this does not actually increase the time required for a consultation (Loh et al. 2007).

Communication style and skills are also important ingredients of a therapeutic alliance. Effective doctor–patient communication is not only clear but also collaborative, involving active listening and a nonauthoritarian orientation to problem solving and conflict resolution (Bultman and Svarstad 2000). Clear and collaborative communication enhances medication adherence (Bultman and Svarstad 2000; Lin et al. 1995). Skilled communication may be especially important in specific populations, such as patients with a dismissive attachment style (Ciechanowski et al. 2001). Discussions regarding medication should have clear explanations of the time course of response and the recommended duration of treatment (Lin et al. 1995). Discussion of anticipated side effects also promotes adherence (Bull et al. 2002). Many of these recommendations border on the obvious but can easily be neglected by harried providers. Less obvious, perhaps, is the finding that adherence is increased when communications to patients with depression involve encouragement to engage in pleasurable activities (Lin et al. 1995; Ströhle 2009).

The Ideal of Patient–Centeredness

At the start of the new millennium, at a time when psychiatry and much of the rest of modern medicine were incorporating more technological efficiencies into the practice of medicine, streamlining the doctor–patient encounter, and increasingly narrowing the focus on symptoms, the Institute of Medicine issued an influential report that addressed major practice gaps in contemporary medicine (Institute of Medicine 2001). One of the six major priorities for American health care that were identified in this report was *patient-centeredness*, defined as "care that is respectful of and responsive to individual patient preferences, needs, and values and ensuring that patient values guide all clinical decisions."

Patient-centeredness, which was initially a psychoanalytic concept coined by the influential Hungarian-British psychoanalyst Michael Balint, has become a mainstream concern not only in psychiatry but in all of medicine. Psychodynamic psychopharmacology is one approach to address this issue. In its essence, psychodynamic psychopharmacology is patient-centered rather than "illness-centered" or "doctor-centered." In an illness-focused (or symptom-focused) approach, according to Enid Balint, "the prime aim is to find a localizable fault, diagnose it as an illness, and then treat it" (E. Balint 1969, p. 269). This approach seems to be the way that American psychiatry has tended to function since the 1990s, with increasing focus on eradicating symptoms and decreased focus on the whole person and on patients' broader developmental aims. In this sense, psychiatrists (or psychopharmacologists, as they now tend to be called) have ceased to be mental health professionals and now function more as mental *illness* professionals. The patient-centered approach of psychodynamic psychopharmacology is one remedy for this problem.

Adopting a patient-centered approach means that "in addition to trying to discover a localizable illness or illnesses, the doctor also has to examine the whole person in order to form what we call an 'overall diagnosis'" (E. Balint 1969, p. 269). The overall diagnosis is Michael Balint's concept for what we now call the "psychodynamic formulation," with a particular emphasis on patients' relationship to treatment and treatment seeking. Balint argued that such a patient-centered approach was especially important in the care of "fat envelope" patients—that is, treatment-resistant patients with thick charts (M. Balint 1957). Psychodynamic psychopharmacology likewise recognizes that, for patients who have failed to benefit from standard, symptom-focused, evidence-based treatments, understanding their relation to illness and treatment is essential to constructing a relationship that marshals their internal resources in the service of recovery.

Patient-centeredness offers a range of benefits to patients, including improved satisfaction with care (Rathert et al. 2013), increased empowerment, and better outcomes (Epstein and Street 2011; Stewart et al. 2000). The health care system benefits as well, because patient-centeredness enhances the efficiency of the system rather than detracting from it. Patient-centered communication, as recommended in psychodynamic psychopharmacology, does not appear to add to the time required for a patient consultation (Epstein et al. 2010; Loh et al. 2007) and is an efficient use of that time. It also seems to create a holding environment (Winnicott 1963) that allows patients and doctors to manage health problems without costly efforts to manage anxiety, such as added laboratory tests or referrals to specialists, thus reducing costs to the system (Stewart et al. 2000). These approaches seem also to benefit doctors in a number of ways. Physicians who adopt a patient-centered practice appear to have a reduced vulnerability to lawsuits (Levinson et al. 1997) and an increased resilience to burnout (Nelson et al. 2014), a problem that is approaching epidemic proportions in American medicine.

Despite the pressures being brought to bear on prescribers to practice in a symptom-focused and biomedically oriented model, a preponderance of evidence suggests psychosocial factors often play a deciding role in whether treatments will work. A patient-centered, psychodynamically informed model such as psychodynamic psychopharmacology offers a framework for treatment that may not only improve clinical outcomes for chronic or treatment-resistant patients but also increase satisfaction on the part of patients and their prescribers.

Key Points

- Pharmacological treatment resistance remains a significant problem in psychiatry despite decades of advances in neurobiology and pharmacotherapy.

- The placebo effect and other meaning and interpersonal effects in pharmacotherapy are potent factors in promoting positive outcomes, often more potent even than medications.

- Patients' character and mindset profoundly shape medication outcomes.

- Prescribers' attitudes, engagement, and prescribing behaviors may determine the effectiveness of pharmacotherapy.

- When treatment resistance emerges from the level of meaning, psychodynamic psychopharmacology provides tools for addressing that resistance.

References

Aikens JE, Kroenke K, Swindle RW, et al: Nine-month predictors and outcomes of SSRI antidepressant continuation in primary care. Gen Hosp Psychiatry 27(4):229–236, 2005 15993253

Aikens JE, Nease DE Jr, Klinkman MS: Explaining patients' beliefs about the necessity and harmfulness of antidepressants. Ann Fam Med 6(1):23–29, 2008 18195311

Ankarberg P, Falkenström F: Treatment of depression with antidepressants is primarily a psychological treatment. Psychotherapy (Chic) 45(3):329–339, 2008 22122494

Bagby RM, Ryder AG, Cristi C: Psychosocial and clinical predictors of response to pharmacotherapy for depression. J Psychiatry Neurosci 27(4):250, 2002

Balint E: The possibilities of patient-centered medicine. J R Coll Gen Pract 17(82):269–276, 1969 5770926

Balint E, Norell JS (eds): Six Minutes for the Patient: Interactions in General Practice Consultation, Vol 2. London, Routledge, 2001

Balint M: The Doctor and His Patient and the Illness. London, Pitman, 1957

Bartholomew K, Horowitz LM: Attachment styles among young adults: a test of a four-category model. J Pers Soc Psychol 61(2):226–244, 1991 1920064

Beitman BD, Beck NC, Deuser WE, et al: Patient stage of change predicts outcome in a panic disorder medication trial. Anxiety 1(2):64–69, 1994 9160550

Bender DS, Skodol AE, Pagano ME, et al: Prospective assessment of treatment use by patients with personality disorders. Psychiatr Serv 57(2):254–257, 2006 16452705

Berlim MT, Turecki G: Definition, assessment, and staging of treatment-resistant refractory major depression: a review of current concepts and methods. Can J Psychiatry 52(1):46–54, 2007 17444078

Blatt SJ, Quinlan DM, Zuroff DC, et al: Interpersonal factors in brief treatment of depression: further analyses of the National Institute of Mental Health Treatment of Depression Collaborative Research Program. J Consult Clin Psychol 64(1):162–171, 1996a 8907096

Blatt SJ, Sanislow CA 3rd, Zuroff DC, et al: Characteristics of effective therapists: further analyses of data from the National Institute of Mental Health Treatment of Depression Collaborative Research Program. J Consult Clin Psychol 64(6):1276–1284, 1996b 8991314

Boudes P: Drug compliance in therapeutic trials: a review. Control Clin Trials 19(3):257–268, 1998 9620809

Bull SA, Hu XH, Hunkeler EM, et al: Discontinuation of use and switching of antidepressants: influence of patient-physician communication. JAMA 288(11):1403–1409, 2002 12234237

Bultman DC, Svarstad BL: Effects of physician communication style on client medication beliefs and adherence with antidepressant treatment. Patient Educ Couns 40(2):173–185, 2000 10771371

Cattaneo AD, Lucchelli PE, Filippucci G: Sedative effects of placebo treatment. Eur J Clin Pharmacol 3:43–45, 1970

Chehil S, Devarajan S, Dursun SM: Pharmacologic management of refractory depression. Can Fam Physician 47:50–52, 2001 11212433

Ciechanowski PS, Katon WJ, Russo JE, et al: The patient-provider relationship: attachment theory and adherence to treatment in diabetes. Am J Psychiatry 158(1):29–35, 2001 11136630

Ciechanowski PS, Russo JE, Katon WJ, et al: The association of patient relationship style and outcomes in collaborative care treatment for depression in patients with diabetes. Med Care 44(3):283–291, 2006 16501401

Clever SL, Ford DE, Rubenstein LV, et al: Primary care patients' involvement in decision-making is associated with improvement in depression. Med Care 44(5):398–405, 2006

Comninos AG, Grenyer BFS: The influence of interpersonal factors on the speed of recovery from major depression. Psychother Res 17(2):230–239, 2007

Cramer JA, Rosenheck R: Compliance with medication regimens for mental and physical disorders. Psychiatr Serv 49(2):196–201, 1998 9575004

Cruz M, Roter DL, Cruz RF, et al: Appointment length, psychiatrists' communication behaviors, and medication management appointment adherence. Psychiatr Serv 64(9):886–892, 2013 23771555

Davis C, Ralevski E, Kennedy SH, et al: The role of personality factors in the reporting of side effect complaints to moclobemide and placebo: a study of healthy male and female volunteers. J Clin Psychopharmacol 15(5):347–352, 1995 8830066

Deacon BJ, Baird GL: The chemical imbalance explanation of depression: reducing blame at what cost? J Soc Clin Psychol 28(4):415–435, 2009

de Craen AJ, Roos PJ, de Vries AL, et al: Effect of colour of drugs: systematic review of perceived effect of drugs and of their effectiveness. BMJ 313(7072):1624–1626, 1996 8991013

de Craen AJ, Tijssen JG, de Gans J, et al: Placebo effect in the acute treatment of migraine: subcutaneous placebos are better than oral placebos. J Neurol 247(3):183–188, 2000 10787112

Downing RW, Rickels K, Dreesmann H: Orthogonal factors vs. interdependent variables as predictors of drug treatment response in anxious outpatients. Psychopharmacology (Berl) 32(2):93–111, 1973 4584949

Dulgar-Tulloch L: An assessment of the positive aspects of depression. Unpublished doctoral dissertation, State University of New York at Albany, 2009

Engel GL: The need for a new medical model: a challenge for biomedicine. Science 196(4286):129–136, 1977 847460

Epstein RM, Street RL Jr: The values and value of patient-centered care. Ann Fam Med 9(2):100–103, 2011 21403134

Epstein RM, Fiscella K, Lesser CS, et al: Why the nation needs a policy push on patient-centered health care. Health Aff (Millwood) 29(8):1489–1495, 2010 20679652

Fast GJ, Fisher S: The role of body attitudes and acquiescence in epinephrine and placebo effects. Psychosom Med 33(1):63–84, 1971 5100735

Fisher S, Greenberg RP (eds): From Placebo to Panacea: Putting Psychiatric Drugs to the Test. Hoboken NJ, Wiley, 1997

Frank E, Kupfer DJ, Siegel LR: Alliance not compliance: a philosophy of outpatient care (discussion). J Clin Psychiatry 56(suppl 1):11–16, discussion 16–17, 1995 7836346

Gaudiano BA, Miller IW: Patients' expectancies, the alliance in pharmacotherapy, and treatment outcomes in bipolar disorder. J Consult Clin Psychol 74(4):671–676, 2006 16881774

Ghaemi SN, Vöhringer PA, Vergne DE: The varieties of depressive experience: diagnosing mood disorders. Psychiatr Clin North Am 35(1):73–86, 2012 22370491

Gutheil TG: The psychology of psychopharmacology. Bull Menninger Clin 46(4):321–330, 1982 7139146

Hahn RA: The nocebo phenomenon: scope and foundations, in The Placebo Effect: An Interdisciplinary Exploration. Edited by Harrington A. Cambridge, MA, Harvard University Press, 1997, pp 56–76

Hollon SD, DeRubeis RJ: Placebo-psychotherapy combinations: inappropriate representations of psychotherapy in drug-psychotherapy comparative trials. Psychol Bull 90(3):467–477, 1981 7029596

Iacoviello BM, McCarthy KS, Barrett MS, et al: Treatment preferences affect the therapeutic alliance: implications for randomized controlled trials. J Consult Clin Psychol 75(1):194–198, 2007 17295580

Institute of Medicine: Crossing the Quality Chasm, A New Health System for the 21st Century. Washington, DC, National Academy Press, 2001

Jaspers K: General Psychopathology [Allgemeine Psychopathologie]. Berlin, Springer, 1913

Jensen KB, Kaptchuk TJ, Kirsch I, et al: Nonconscious activation of placebo and nocebo pain responses. Proc Natl Acad Sci U S A 109(39):15959–15964, 2012 23019380

Joyce PR, Paykel ES: Predictors of drug response in depression. Arch Gen Psychiatry 46(1):89–99, 1989 2562916

Kaplan JE, Keeley RD, Engel M, et al: Aspects of patient and clinician language predict adherence to antidepressant medication. J Am Board Fam Med 26(4):409–420, 2013 23833156

Kaptchuk TJ, Goldman P, Stone DA, et al: Do medical devices have enhanced placebo effects? J Clin Epidemiol 53(8):786–792, 2000 10942860

Kemp JJ, Lickel JJ, Deacon BJ: Effects of a chemical imbalance causal explanation on individuals' perceptions of their depressive symptoms. Behav Res Ther 56:47–52, 2014 24657311

Kennedy WP: The nocebo reaction. Med World 95:203–205, 1961 13752532

Kessler RC, Berglund P, Demler O, et al: The epidemiology of major depressive disorder: results from the National Comorbidity Survey Replication (NCS-R). JAMA 289(23):3095–3105, 2003 12813115

Khan A, Warner HA, Brown WA: Symptom reduction and suicide risk in patients treated with placebo in antidepressant clinical trials: an analysis of the Food and Drug Administration database. Arch Gen Psychiatry 57(4):311–317, 2000 10768687

Khan A, Redding N, Brown WA: The persistence of the placebo response in antidepressant clinical trials. J Psychiatr Res 42(10):791–796, 2008 18036616

Kirsch I, Sapirstein G: Listening to Prozac but hearing placebo: a meta-analysis of antidepressant medication. Prevention and Treatment 1(2), 1998

Kirsch I, Mearns J, Catanzaro SJ: Mood-regulation expectancies as determinants of dysphoria in college students. J Couns Psychol 37(3):306, 1990

Kirsch I, Moore TJ, Scoboria A, et al: The emperor's new drugs: an analysis of antidepressant medication data submitted to the U.S. Food and Drug Administration. Prevention and Treatment 5(23)453–462, 2002

Kocsis JH, Leon AC, Markowitz JC, et al: Patient preference as a moderator of outcome for chronic forms of major depressive disorder treated with nefazodone, cognitive behavioral analysis system of psychotherapy, or their combination. J Clin Psychiatry 70(3):354–361, 2009 19192474

Krell HV, Leuchter AF, Morgan M, et al: Subject expectations of treatment effectiveness and outcome of treatment with an experimental antidepressant. J Clin Psychiatry 65(9):1174–1179, 2004 15367043

Kronström K, Salminen JK, Hietala J, et al: Does defense style or psychological mindedness predict treatment response in major depression? Depress Anxiety 26(7):689–695, 2009 19496102

Krupnick JL, Sotsky SM, Simmens S, et al: The role of the therapeutic alliance in psychotherapy and pharmacotherapy outcome: findings in the National Institute of Mental Health Treatment of Depression Collaborative Research Program. J Consult Clin Psychol 64(3):532–539, 1996 8698947

Kwan BM, Dimidjian S, Rizvi SL: Treatment preference, engagement, and clinical improvement in pharmacotherapy versus psychotherapy for depression. Behav Res Ther 48(8):799–804, 2010 20462569

Lebowitz MS, Ahn WK, Nolen-Hoeksema S: Fixable or fate? Perceptions of the biology of depression. J Consult Clin Psychol 81(3):518–527, 2013 23379262

Levinson W, Roter DL, Mullooly JP, et al: Physician-patient communication: the relationship with malpractice claims among primary care physicians and surgeons. JAMA 277(7):553–559, 1997 9032162

Lewis CC, Simons AD, Silva SG, et al: The role of readiness to change in response to treatment of adolescent depression. J Consult Clin Psychol 77(3):422–428, 2009 19485584

Lieberman JA, Stroup TS, McEvoy JP, et al: Effectiveness of antipsychotic drugs in patients with chronic schizophrenia. N Engl J Med 353(12):1209–1223, 2005 16172203

Lin EH, Von Korff M, Katon W, et al: The role of the primary care physician in patients' adherence to antidepressant therapy. Med Care 33(1):67–74, 1995 7823648

Lin P, Campbell DG, Chaney EF, et al: The influence of patient preference on depression treatment in primary care. Ann Behav Med 30(2):164–173, 2005 16173913

Loh A, Simon D, Wills CE, et al: The effects of a shared decision-making intervention in primary care of depression: a cluster-randomized controlled trial. Patient Educ Couns 67(3):324–332, 2007 17509808

Lyerly SB, Ross S, Krugman AD, et al: Drugs and placebos: the effects of instructions upon performance and mood under amphetamine sulfate and chloral hydrate. J Abnorm Psychol 68(3):321–327, 1964 14126847

Mayberg HS, Silva JA, Brannan SK, et al: The functional neuroanatomy of the placebo effect. Am J Psychiatry 159(5):728–737, 2002 11986125

McKay KM, Imel ZE, Wampold BE: Psychiatrist effects in the psychopharmacological treatment of depression. J Affect Disord 92(2–3):287–290, 2006 16503356

McNair DM, Kahn RJ, Droppelman RF, et al: Compatibility, acquiescence, and drug effects, in Neuro-Psycho-Pharmacology: Proceedings of the Fifth International Congress of the Collegium Internationale Neuro-Psycho Pharmacologicum. Edited by Brill H. New York, Excerpta Medica Foundation, 1968, pp 536–542

McNair DM, Fisher S, Kahn RJ, et al: Drug-personality interaction in intensive outpatient treatment. Arch Gen Psychiatry 22(2):128–135, 1970 4903499

Meyer B, Pilkonis PA, Krupnick JL, et al: Treatment expectancies, patient alliance, and outcome: further analyses from the National Institute of Mental Health Treatment of Depression Collaborative Research Program. J Consult Clin Psychol 70(4):1051–1055, 2002 12182269

Mintz D: Meaning and medication in the care of treatment-resistant patients. Am J Psychother 56(3):322–337, 2002 12400200

Mintz D, Belnap B: A view from Riggs—treatment resistance and patient authority, III: what is psychodynamic psychopharmacology? An approach to pharmacologic treatment resistance. J Am Acad Psychoanal Dyn Psychiatry 34(4):581–601, 2006 17274730

Mintz DL, Belnap B: What is psychodynamic psychopharmacology? An approach to pharmacological treatment resistance, in Treatment Resistance and Patient Authority: The Austen Riggs Reader. Edited by Plakun E. New York, WW Norton, 2011, pp 42–65

Nelson KM, Helfrich C, Sun H, et al: Implementation of the patient-centered medical home in the Veterans Health Administration: associations with patient satisfaction, quality of care, staff burnout, and hospital and emergency department use. JAMA Intern Med 174(8):1350–1358, 2014 25055197

Perlis RH, Ostacher MJ, Patel JK, et al: Predictors of recurrence in bipolar disorder: primary outcomes from the Systematic Treatment Enhancement Program for Bipolar Disorder (STEP-BD). Am J Psychiatry 163(2):217–224, 2006 16449474

Peselow ED, Robins CJ, Sanfilipo MP, et al: Sociotropy and autonomy: relationship to antidepressant drug treatment response and endogenous-nonendogenous dichotomy. J Abnorm Psychol 101(3):479–486, 1992 1386856

Piguet V, Cedraschi C, Dumont P, et al: Patients' representations of antidepressants: a clue to nonadherence? Clin J Pain 23(8):669–675, 2007 17885345

Plakun EM: A view from Riggs—treatment resistance and patient authority, I: a psychodynamic perspective on treatment resistance. J Am Acad Psychoanal Dyn Psychiatry 34(2):349–366, 2006 16780414

Plakun EM: Psychodynamic psychiatry, the biopsychosocial model, and the difficult patient. Psychiatr Clin North Am 41(2):237–248, 2018 29739523

Pound P, Britten N, Morgan M, et al: Resisting medicines: a synthesis of qualitative studies of medicine taking. Soc Sci Med 61(1):133–155, 2005 15847968

Rathert C, Wyrwich MD, Boren SA: Patient-centered care and outcomes: a systematic review of the literature. Med Care Res Rev 70(4):351–379, 2013 23169897

Raue PJ, Schulberg HC, Heo M, et al: Patients' depression treatment preferences and initiation, adherence, and outcome: a randomized primary care study. Psychiatr Serv 60(3):337–343, 2009 19252046

Reynaert C, Janne P, Vause M, et al: Clinical trials of antidepressants: the hidden face: where locus of control appears to play a key role in depression outcome. Psychopharmacology (Berl) 119(4):449–454, 1995 7480525

Rickels K, Lipman RS, Park LC, et al: Drug, doctor warmth, and clinic setting in the symptomatic response to minor tranquilizers. Psychopharmacology (Berl) 20(2):128–152, 1971 4933093

Rogers A: Star neuroscientist Tom Insel leaves the Google-spawned Verily for…a startup. Wired, 2017. Available at: www.wired.com/2017/05/star-neuroscientist-tom-insel-leaves-google-spawned-verily-startup. Accessed May 25, 2021.

Roman B: Patients' attitudes towards generic substitution of oral atypical antipsychotics. CNS Drugs 23(8):693–701, 2009

Rosen DC, Nakash O, Alegría M: The impact of computer use on therapeutic alliance and continuance in care during the mental health intake. Psychotherapy (Chic) 53(1):117–123, 2016 26214322

Rotter JB: Generalized expectancies for internal versus external control of reinforcement. Psychol Monogr Gen Appl 80(1):1–28, 1966 5340840

Rush AJ, Thase ME: Improving depression outcome by patient-centered medical management. Am J Psychiatry 175(12):1187–1198, 2018 30220219

Rutherford BR, Wager TD, Roose SP: Expectancy and the treatment of depression: a review of experimental methodology and effects on patient outcome. Curr Psychiatry Rev 6(1):1–10, 2010 24812548

Schapira K, McClelland HA, Griffiths NR, et al: Study on the effects of tablet colour in the treatment of anxiety states. BMJ 1(5707):446–449, 1970 5420207

Scott J, Williams JM, Brittlebank A, et al: The relationship between premorbid neuroticism, cognitive dysfunction and persistence of depression: a 1-year follow-up. J Affect Disord 33(3):167–172, 1995 7790668

Sirey JA, Bruce ML, Alexopoulos GS, et al: Stigma as a barrier to recovery: perceived stigma and patient-rated severity of illness as predictors of antidepressant drug adherence. Psychiatr Serv 52(12):1615–1620, 2001 11726752

Skodol AE, Gunderson JG, Shea MT, et al: The Collaborative Longitudinal Personality Disorders Study (CLPS): overview and implications. J Pers Disord 19(5):487–504, 2005 16274278

Skodol AE, Grilo CM, Keyes KM, et al: Relationship of personality disorders to the course of major depressive disorder in a nationally representative sample. Am J Psychiatry 168(3):257–264, 2011 21245088

Sneed JR, Rutherford BR, Rindskopf D, et al: Design makes a difference: a meta-analysis of antidepressant response rates in placebo-controlled versus comparator trials in late-life depression. Am J Geriatr Psychiatry 16(1):65–73, 2008 17998306

Squier RW: A model of empathic understanding and adherence to treatment regimens in practitioner-patient relationships. Soc Sci Med 30(3):325–339, 1990 2408150

Steunenberg B, Beekman AT, Deeg DJ, et al: Personality predicts recurrence of late-life depression. J Affect Disord 123(1–3):164–172, 2010 19758704

Stewart M, Brown JB, Donner A, et al: The impact of patient-centered care on outcomes. J Fam Pract 49(9):796–804, 2000 11032203

Ströhle A: Physical activity, exercise, depression and anxiety disorders. J Neural Transm (Vienna) 116(6):777–784, 2009 18726137

Sullivan MD, Katon WJ, Russo JE, et al: Patient beliefs predict response to paroxetine among primary care patients with dysthymia and minor depression. J Am Board Fam Pract 16(1):22–31, 2003 12583647

Thase ME, Friedman ES, Howland RH: Management of treatment-resistant depression: psychotherapeutic perspectives. J Clin Psychiatry 62(suppl 18):18–24, 2001 11575731

Thase ME, Friedman ES, Biggs MM, et al: Cognitive therapy versus medication in augmentation and switch strategies as second-step treatments: a STAR*D report. Am J Psychiatry 164(5):739–752, 2007 17475733

Treloar AJ: Effectiveness of education programs in changing clinicians' attitudes toward treating borderline personality disorder. Psychiatr Serv 60(8):1128–1131, 2009 19648203

Uhlenhuth EH, Rickels K, Fisher S, et al: Drug, doctor's verbal attitude and clinic setting in the symptomatic response to pharmacotherapy. Psychopharmacology (Berl) 9(5):392–418, 1966 4872909

van Egmond J, Kummeling I: A blind spot for secondary gain affecting therapy outcomes. Eur Psychiatry 17(1):46–54, 2002 11918993

van Egmond J, Kummeling I, Balkom TA: Secondary gain as hidden motive for getting psychiatric treatment. Eur Psychiatry 20(5–6):416–421, 2005 16171656

Waber RL, Shiv B, Carmon Z, et al: Commercial features of placebo and therapeutic efficacy. JAMA 299(9):1016–1017, 2008 18319411

Warden D, Trivedi MH, Wisniewski SR, et al: Identifying risk for attrition during treatment for depression. Psychother Psychosom 78(6):372–379, 2009 19738403

Weissenfeld J, Stock S, Lüngen M, et al: The nocebo effect: a reason for patients' nonadherence to generic substitution? Pharmazie 65(7):451–456, 2010 20662309

Westen D, Morrison K: A multidimensional meta-analysis of treatments for depression, panic, and generalized anxiety disorder: an empirical examination of the status of empirically supported therapies. J Consult Clin Psychol 69(6):875–899, 2001 11777114

Williams LM, Debattista C, Duchemin AM, et al: Childhood trauma predicts antidepressant response in adults with major depression: data from the randomized international study to predict optimized treatment for depression. Transl Psychiatry 6(5):e799, 2016

Winnicott D: Psychiatric disorders in terms of infantile maturational processes, in The Maturational Process and the Facilitating Environment. New York, International Universities Press, 1963, pp 230–240

Woolley SB, Fredman L, Goethe JW, et al: Hospital patients' perceptions during treatment and early discontinuation of serotonin selective reuptake inhibitor antidepressants. J Clin Psychopharmacol 30(6):716–719, 2010 21105288

Zuroff DC, Koestner R, Moskowitz DS, et al: Autonomous motivation for therapy: a new common factor in brief treatments for depression. Psychother Res 17(2):137–147, 2007

CHAPTER 3

What Is Psychodynamic About Psychodynamic Psychopharmacology?

Words are, of course, the most powerful drug used by mankind.

—Rudyard Kipling, speech to the Royal College
of Surgeons in London, 1923

Psychodynamic psychopharmacology, may, at some point, have sounded like an oxymoron because psychodynamic psychiatry and biomedical psychiatry seemed to be pitted against one another. Although psychoanalysis, especially as practiced in the United States in mid-20th century, tended to disparage biomedical psychiatry as a mere Band-Aid, this was not at all the vision held by Sigmund Freud. Freud saw himself as a biomedical psychiatrist, and he saw his technique as making adjustments to the hormonal and nervous systems of his patients. He was well aware that psychiatry was in its infancy. He did not at all see the "talking cure" as the be-all and end-all of psychiatry but, rather, as the best available option at the time. With uncharacteristic optimism, he noted in 1926: "We may look forward to a day when paths of knowledge and, let us hope, influence will be opened up, leading from organized biology and chemistry to the field of neurotic phenomena" (Freud 1926/1959, p. 231). Over a decade later, in the last year of his life, he envisioned, without any sense of disparagement or competitiveness, the advent of psychopharmacology: "The future may teach us to exercise a direct influence, by means of particular substances, on the amounts of energy and their distribution in the mental apparatus. It may be that there are still undreamt-of possibilities of therapy" (Freud 1940[1938]/1964, p. 182).

Even as he recognized that medications might someday more efficiently and effectively address the neurotic suffering that was the purview of psychoanalysis, Freud did not envision that psychoanalysis would become obsolete. Instead, he saw a synergy between psychoanalysis and psychopharmacology (or, in his day, endocrinology) in which the analyst, with an understanding of the patient's unconscious conflicts, would be able to help the prescriber more effectively target psychiatric treatments.

> In hospitals like this, the cooperation of psychoanalysts and other clinicians will make it possible to study the relationship between psychic and somatic processes. Through the collaboration of psychoanalysts, I look forward to an important contribution to endocrinology. It is possible that the endocrinologists may find out more and more what psychic changes may occur as a consequence of changes in the hormonic tone. I, therefore, believe it possible that endocrinologists may, after they have gained more knowledge and technique, succeed in producing direct psychic changes....Even then, the psychoanalyst will probably not be superfluous. On the basis of his knowledge of processes within the unconscious he will probably be able to give the endocrinologist suggestions for hormontherapeutic measures. (Sigmund Freud to Professor Becker, Prussian Minister of Art, Science, and Education, as quoted in Simmel 1937, pp. 141–142)

In this spirit, psychodynamic psychopharmacology aims to help elucidate psychological and interpersonal dynamics that can either interfere with or promote optimal response to pharmacotherapy. Acting as a complement to rational pharmacotherapy, an in-depth understanding of the patient can help the prescriber recognize what psychosocial factors may be impacting that patient's unique medication response. In this way, the prescriber not only has a framework for *what* medication to prescribe but also *how* to engage with the patient to minimize resistance and optimize the psychological factors that are concordant with the desired psychopharmacological effect.

In many ways, psychodynamic psychopharmacology extends recognition of the important role that common factors, such as an emotionally charged confiding relationship, a therapeutic rationale, provision of new information, and instillation of hope, play in all psychiatric interventions (Frank 1971), including both psychotherapy and psychopharmacotherapy. In its approach, however, psychodynamic psychopharmacology conceptualizes these factors from a psychodynamic perspective. For example, although acknowledging that the alliance is a crucial factor for pharmacotherapy outcome, a psychodynamic perspective considers that the alliance is itself affected by a range of factors, including transferences based on past experiences, unconscious and unexpressed wishes and ideas about treatment (from both patient and prescriber), and related notions.

Table 3–1.   Key psychodynamic concepts relevant to pharmacotherapy

Attachment style
Conflict or ambivalence
Defense
Resistance
Transference
The unconscious

Basic Psychodynamics Impacting Medication Responsiveness

Psychodynamic psychopharmacology is founded on a view of psychological functioning that draws from many of the fundamental insights of psychoanalysis (Table 3–1). Most fundamentally, it begins with an understanding of people as being motivated by complex and conflicting dynamics. *Psychodynamic* refers to a conceptualization of mental life as a roiling amalgamation of individuals' desires, impulses, fears, and values. These are frequently at cross-purposes, with some coming to the fore directly, others emerging in the form of a compromise between competing impulses, and still others suppressed and then expressed surreptitiously in some disguised form. In this view, conscious mental life represents a compromise among these differing mental forces. The essentially conflictual nature of mental life means patients will always be ambivalent about the care they receive. In any given moment, patients are likely to be struggling with multiple competing agendas. Depending on the force of the various trends toward or away from recovery, they will be more or less prone to respond positively to treatment.

Manifestly, patients seek care for psychiatric symptoms and may seem to set recovery as a priority. Beneath this, however, they may have temporarily been relieved of onerous responsibilities by virtue of the sick role (Parsons 1951). For example, their symptoms may carry hidden gratifications, such as relative permission to behave in a regressive, dependent, or demanding way, as long as it is thought of as a symptom. At the same time, by virtue of early caregiving experiences, patients may harbor resentment and suspicion of authority figures in a caregiving role. People who have experienced early adversity often automatically distrust and resist authority, including medical authority. More deeply still, they may be motivated by a desire for love and have found that their illness gives them access to caregiving that would otherwise be unavailable, so they stand to lose something important if they recover. One of the pharmacologist's core tasks is to identify and work with each patient's ambivalence and, in doing so, help manage these resistances, both conscious and unconscious, and optimize outcomes.

Drawing further from the fundamental insights of psychoanalysis, psychodynamic psychopharmacology recognizes that many of the processes that contribute to treatment resistance are largely unconscious for patients (and prescribers), occurring beyond their awareness but influencing their behavior nonetheless. An example of one aspect of the unconscious is *implicit social cognitions* (Greenwald and Banaji 1995), or lessons a person has learned so basically that they fundamentally shape and filter that person's experience without the person even being aware of it. Furthermore, the *dynamic unconscious* ostensibly contains those thoughts that are kept out of awareness by an internal censor because they fundamentally clash with the person's ideals, self-image, or other important aspects of conscious awareness.

Regarding pharmacotherapy, patients who are ambivalent about their recovery may have little awareness of countertherapeutic trends in their mental life. Consciously, they want to get better and may be genuinely puzzled by their difficulty remembering to take medications or their participation in other treatment-interfering illness behaviors. Similarly, patients who are prone to nocebo responses may be legitimately unaware of the expectations of harm that predispose them to be harmed by medications (Jensen et al. 2012). One implication of this understanding is a paradoxical recognition of the ways patients may be seen as responsible but not blameworthy for their treatment resistance. Part of the task of the prescriber, like that of the psychodynamic psychotherapist, is to work with patients in such a way that their unconscious becomes conscious. Only when the countertherapeutic aspects of a patient's psychology become conscious can that patient begin to gain control over these tendencies.

Another implication of a psychodynamic perspective on prescribing is an understanding that our conscious mental life is shaped by myriad defense mechanisms (explored in depth in Chapter 4) whose purpose is to manage the roiling, conflictual nature of the mind. Indeed, defense mechanisms protect the self from the disorganizing pressure of so many competing demands and preserve an idealized sense of self by keeping distressing realizations out of awareness. Although they are crucial aspects of the psyche, defense mechanisms may also keep individuals from recognizing the nature or the seriousness of their troubles. For example, patients with psychotic illness may acquiesce to grandiosity and resist treatment precisely because it is too painful to face the devastating consequences of their illness and the profound loneliness that often accompanies severe psychiatric illness.

Defensive operations, conversely, may also lead patients to attach to diagnoses and treatments in unhelpful ways in an effort to avoid feelings of responsibility, guilt, and shame. One example is the patient who explains all interpersonally destructive behavior as the result of "my bipolar," essentially making her behaviors the doctor's responsibility because he has failed to find the right medications to contain them. Although patients who rely on this defensive maneuver may feel instantly relieved, they invariably do worse in the long term because the medical defense absolves them of responsibility, giving free rein to their destructive impulses. Until the prescriber (or therapist) can appreciate how psychopharmacotherapy interacts with defenses, such countertherapeutic factors will operate freely, interfering with optimal outcomes.

Another central psychodynamic concept is the phenomenon of *transference*, which can be understood as the tendency to experience current relationships as echoes of past relationships. We learn our most basic lessons about what others are like within the context of our early relationships. Typically, these formative experiences occur within our family of origin and then become a filter through which we experience other relationships. Transference dynamics invariably emerge in the prescribing relationship even if they are not directly acknowledged and attended to by the prescriber. However, if appropriately recognized and engaged, transference-based expectations provide important opportunities for the prescribing relationship. Indeed, patients often have a history of early adversity that complicates the working alliance and treatment outcome. For example, a patient with self-preoccupied and neglectful parents often expects prescribers to be unreliable and primarily focused on their own needs. Even minor evidence of inattention or self-interest on the part of a prescriber then confirms this patient's transference expectations, undermining a solid alliance that might have supported good treatment outcomes. On the other hand, patients who experienced reliable and competent parenting are likely to have more positive transferences to caregiving, promoting a solid working alliance and amplifying beneficial effects from positive treatment expectancies.

Attachment styles (Ainsworth and Bell 1970; Bowlby 1958, 1973), like transference dynamics, also shape treatment outcomes. Attachment styles can be understood as enduring patterns of self-and-other experience (Bartholomew and Horowitz 1991) that determine our future relational patterns (Table 3–2). When early relational experiences allow a child to develop positive views of both the self and others, that child grows to have a capacity for secure attachments. Patients with generally reliable, emotionally attuned, and benevolent early caregiving tend to develop secure attachments. Securely attached people tend to have positive views of themselves and others and feel comfortable with both intimacy and independence in those relationships. Furthermore, securely attached people are more likely to view their relationships as satisfactory (Sable 2008) than people with other attachment styles.

Table 3–2.   Attachment styles and pharmacotherapy

	View of self	
	Positive	Negative
Positive View of other **Negative**	*Secure* Comfortable with intimacy and autonomy Trusting of providers Retains sense of self-efficacy *Dismissing* Dismissing of intimacy Counterdependent Gives up on treatments quickly Takes treatment matters into their own hands	*Preoccupied* Preoccupied with relationships May be acquiescent or dependent in treatment relationships Needs frequent reassurance or support *Fearful* Fearful of intimacy Socially avoidant Expects to be harmed Prone to nocebo responses

Source.   Adapted from the attachment matrix of Bartholomew and Horowitz 1991.

These patients find it easier to develop healthy and balanced relationships with their significant others, health care providers, and medications (Bennett et al. 2011; Ciechanowski et al. 2004; Tyrrell et al. 1999) and often respond more quickly to pharmacotherapy, at least in terms of antidepressant treatment (Comninos and Grenyer 2007).

Patients with less-than-optimal early caregiving experiences are more likely to form attachments in which there are problems with closeness, trust, and dependency. Patients with an anxious-preoccupied attachment style, in general, describe early caregiving experiences as inconsistent and benevolent when available. When care is not available, they typically fault themselves because they have a generally negative sense of self and a positive sense of the other. As a consequence, they strive to get as much caregiving as possible and may become quite dependent. Such patients are likely to work hard to please their doctors if an emotional attachment occurs. On a deeper level, however, they may resist becoming well if it means losing a cherished and predictable source of caring, such as from mental health professionals. These patients, by virtue of their characterological acquiescence, may also be more prone to experience side effects.

Patients with experiences of more actively harmful or critical caregiving are predisposed to develop a fearful-avoidant attachment style. Although they want relationships, they have a fundamental expectation that they will get hurt and a generally negative view of both the self and others. As such, these patients are somewhat chaotic in their relationships, seeking closeness but then also fleeing the dangers of intimacy. They have difficulty trusting others and are uncomfortable in positions of dependency. This may manifest in the doctor–patient relationship as approach-avoidance struggles that impact attendance, quiet control struggles, and nocebo responsiveness often stemming from expectations of harm, among other complications.

Patients with early caregiving experiences that are reliably unreliable tend to develop a dismissive attachment style. These patients, comprising about 11% of the population in nonclinical samples, expect little from others and prefer to depend on themselves. These "one strike and you're out" patients do not tolerate disappointing caregiving. Easily giving up on care providers and on other people in their lives, they "throw out the baby with the bathwater" and give up on treatments. Such patients have been shown to adhere less to medications and to behavioral recommendations for disease management (Ciechanowski et al. 2004). However, these adverse effects of attachment style may be nullified if the patient experiences the treater as providing good communication (Ciechanowski et al. 2001).

The psychoanalytic concept of object relations is also quite relevant to the practice of psychodynamic psychopharmacology. Object relations theory takes the concept of transference one step further, suggesting that early caregiver experiences not only impact the way people relate to others but also fundamentally shape the way people relate to themselves. For example, a child with a harsh and punitive parent may incorporate that aspect of the parent into the self, developing a harsh and punitive superego. These internalized object relations then become the basic models of how the patient experiences the self and others, including the prescriber.

Medications may also function as objects (Tutter 2006). Beyond stereotypical symbolic representations based on the mode of oral incorporation (e.g., medications as nourishment or poison), medications may develop very idiosyncratic meanings based on patients' early experiences and relational models. They may come to represent important others or parts of the self based on internalized object relationships. The medications may come to serve important emotional functions, such as soothing (e.g., a patient who experiences an opiate concretely as a warm embrace), or be experienced as controlling or even punitive. The nature of patients' relationship with medications, conscious and unconscious, shapes a range of factors, including their willingness to take the medications (or not), the nature of their clinical response, and their tendency to experience side effects.

Prescribers must be attentive to psychological factors in patients that run counter to the intent of treatment. Addressing these factors requires, in some cases, that prescribers behave differently (e.g., emphasizing good communication with patients who have a dismissive attachment style and attending to and directly engaging ruptures in the treatment relationship). In other cases, prescribers may help patients change countertherapeutic attitudes and beliefs by helping them become aware of unconscious resistances to treatment and make a conscious choice about how to engage treatment. However, the work of making the unconscious conscious is not so simple as showing it to patients once. Patients often resist treaters' efforts to bring unconscious countertherapeutic factors to awareness and to shift the patients' dynamic toward a healthier adaptation. Having worked hard to achieve some equilibrium by carefully, albeit unconsciously, crafting a compromise between their many competing and conflicting impulses, patients are often deeply frightened to relinquish these solutions. The process of "working through" these resistances is helped by recognizing that the process takes time, empathically recognizing the difficulty involved in giving up defensive positions, and having a capacity for perseverance.

The Concept of Authority

Psychodynamically informed attitudes are as central to the practice of psychodynamic psychopharmacology as psychodynamic concepts. Foremost among these is the notion of patient authority. Whereas a biologically reductive approach tends to view patients as victims of their genes or of "chemical imbalance," psychodynamic psychopharmacologists are more likely to see patients as also having agency. This includes some capacity to influence the course of illness, for better or worse. Again, this is not to say that there is not a major biological component (Cooper 1985) to psychiatric illness, but rather, that patients' relationship with their illness shapes their outcome.

Regardless of how "biological" a problem is, patients have internal resources that can be recruited to address the problems they face. Although sources of inner strength may be drawn on to facilitate treatment, they may also be mobilized in ways that, although intended to solve some problem, actually undercut treatment efforts. For example, patients may recruit symptoms to address defensive needs or to solve interpersonal conflicts, creating reasons to resist treatment. On the other hand, patients may become active participants in recovery, adopting attitudes and behaviors that can support (or even replace) pharmacotherapy. For example, a patient with bipolar disorder may learn to function as his or her own mood stabilizer by focusing effort on developing healthy social rhythms that contribute to a stable mood. In this way, the patient is not a passive battleground between the doctor and the disease but an important ally or adversary in the fight. These dynamics and the ways in which they are engaged invariably impact the outcome of pharmacological treatment.

This position in relation to patient authority has implications for the nature of the therapeutic alliance. Alliance, first of all, is not simply treatment compliance—as in the biomedical alliance (Gutheil and Havens 1979), in which the doctor is the expert on what medications are appropriate for which symptoms or diagnoses. In psychodynamic psychopharmacology, prescribers *cannot* assume that eradication of symptoms is their patients' primary goal. Patients may place a premium on the feeling of autonomy, on the opportunity to be cared for in the sick role, or on being able to differentiate which aspects of improvement are caused by medications and which are the result of their efforts. Prescribers may be the experts on what medications are appropriate for specific symptoms, but patients remain the experts on their own treatment goals. As in a psychotherapeutic contract, the alliance is based on reasonable goals established by patients and collaboratively negotiated with prescribers.

In an effort to authorize patients, however, psychodynamically informed prescribers must also understand that patients' authority has limits. Distinct from recovery-oriented prescribing (Baker et al. 2013)—in which there is an intention to fully empower patients, partly as compensation for the history of disempowering mental health consumers—a psychodynamic psychopharmacologist appreciates that patients' authority is bounded by the unconscious. To the extent that patients are driven by unconscious motivations, they cannot truly be in charge and need the help of others. In this sense, full authority is something for which one strives but does not achieve in the work of trying to bring the unconscious into consciousness. The psychopharmacologist (and therapist) must broaden and deepen patients' authority by trying to notice and bring to light unconscious aspects of their relationship with medications and treatment so that they can then make conscious decisions about how to engage (or not engage) in treatment.

However, the limitations on authority posed by the unconscious cut both ways; patients are not the only ones in the doctor–patient relationship who have an unconscious. Like their patients, doctors cannot know the extent to which their own decision making and orientation to their patients is rational or is influenced by unconscious factors. Patients, especially those who are likely to be treatment refractory, often engender a range of strong feelings in doctors that, whether helplessness, anger, or love, fuel rescue fantasies and shape how those doctors approach those patients. Indeed, in the case of more primitively organized patients, medical decision making may be primarily guided by irrationality (Waldinger and Frank 1989). Like patients, prescribers also cannot be fully in charge of themselves and need the help of others to recognize when they are being led astray from rational prescribing by irrational and unconscious factors. To do this, they must first be aware that the act of prescribing may be suffused with irrationality and attempt to attune themselves to the places in which they have deviated from usual practice patterns or in which vague feelings of discomfort (e.g., shame) shine a light on irrational aspects of pharmacotherapy. In such cases, it can be useful to consult with peers who are not embedded in the same transference-countertransference matrix with the patient and thus are free from the same unconscious emotional pressures.

Perhaps more important, prescribers may turn to patients to illuminate unconscious processes, just as the patients turn to the prescribers. When a patient offers a criticism, the prescriber must preserve a place beyond defensiveness to seriously consider the question of "how is the patient right" (Shapiro 2019). Considering this question is an effective way for prescribers to begin to see what has previously been out of their awareness. Involving patients in medical decision-making processes is another way for prescribers to contain the effects of their own irrationality on the medication regimen. Evidence suggests that involving patients in medical decision making leads to treatments that are more, not less, concordant with treatment guidelines (Clever et al. 2006). Given the role that irrationality plays for both patients and doctors, a good alliance is one in which there is at least a tacit recognition that the relationship is interdependent.

Essentials of Psychodynamic Treatment

Psychodynamic psychopharmacology not only incorporates ideas central to psychoanalysis, such as those of the unconscious or of internal conflict, into patients' understanding but also incorporates psychodynamic attitudes and techniques into the clinical work. Although the specific techniques are elucidated in later chapters, the question may still be raised about what, in the clinical process of psychodynamic psychopharmacology, is *psychodynamic*. What specific types of behaviors differentiate psychodynamic work from other approaches? In their empirical study of therapeutic characteristics that differentiate psychodynamic from cognitive-behavioral approaches, Blagys and Hilsenroth (2000) identified seven features of psychotherapy that were distinct to and characteristic of psychodynamic psychotherapy:

1. Focuses on affect and the expression of patients' emotions
2. Explores patients' attempts to avoid topics or to engage in activities that hinder the progress of therapy
3. Identifies patterns in patients' actions, thoughts, feelings, experiences, and relationships

4. Emphasizes past experiences
5. Focuses on interpersonal experiences
6. Emphasizes the therapeutic relationship
7. Explores patients' wishes, dreams, and fantasies

Although psychodynamic psychopharmacology is not psychotherapy proper, psychotherapeutic skills are utilized in the service of understanding treatment-resistant patients' relationship to treatment and medications and in addressing psychological resistances to the healthy use of medications.

Focus on Affect and the Expression of Patients' Emotions

A focus on affect and on patients' expression of emotions is important in psychodynamic psychopharmacology in several ways. First, to the extent that practitioners are focused on identifying less conscious aspects of patients' experiences of treatment, it is helpful to attend to subtle shifts in their affect and to bring these to their attention. For example, noticing a subtle increase in anxiety or defensiveness in a patient may bring sources of resistance to treatment into awareness. Second, for patients who have given themselves over to a medical system of meaning in which emotions are interpreted primarily through a diagnostic lens, focusing on their understanding of their emotions may help them begin to sort out the complicated question of problems of living versus problems of illness (B. Belnap, personal communication, 2010). Patients who have a highly biologized view of their troubles may need help understanding that their bad feelings not only may be signs of pathology but also may be normal and healthy signals of problems that need to be addressed. Helping them register and organize feelings in this way can help both patients and prescribers to differentiate which forms of suffering might call for medication and which are better to acknowledge, bear, and work through.

Explore Patients' Attempts to Avoid Topics or Engage in Activities That Hinder the Progress of Therapy

In psychodynamic psychotherapy, patients' avoidance of topics often points precisely to issues that are most problematic in their mental life. When a patient announces at the beginning of therapy that she is "not going to talk about my sister," the therapist recognizes that this eventually will become an important topic, and the avoidance will have to be understood. Similarly, if a patient entering treatment announces that he does not want to talk about specific medications or classes of medications, the pharmacotherapist knows that this issue is likely to be quite meaningful. In psychodynamic psycho-pharmacology, exploration of patients' avoidance behaviors may be limited to understanding why they exclude certain medications from consideration, understanding issues of nonadherence, and understanding the problems that underlie missed appointments. Psychodynamic psychopharmacologists also explore the defensive functions of medications (discussed in the chapters that follow) that interfere with patients' authority, adaptability, and medication responsiveness.

Identify Patterns in Patients' Actions, Thoughts, Feelings, Experiences, and Relationships

As part of the effort to address sources of treatment resistance, psychodynamic psychopharmacologists will, from the beginning of treatment, consider how attending to patterns in their patients' lives may help identify sources of their pharmacological treatment resistance. Often, the relational paradigms that drive these patterns also show up in the patients' relationship with their doctor or more directly in the patients' relationship with medications. For example, a patient who has struggled to form stable relationships because of her strong need for control is likely to find that control struggles are also a feature of pharmacological treatment, and her refusal to be controlled may manifest as nonadherence. A prescriber who has inquired about and listened for such patterns will recognize that addressing these struggles by asserting power over the patient is likely to backfire. On the other hand, if these dynamics can be identified and made conscious, the doctor and patient will have an opportunity to address the underlying difficulty. This level of engagement is likely to lead to more collaborative and even transformative outcomes as the patient encounters less resistance to the medication or prescriber and new experiences with a caregiver.

Emphasize Past Experiences

A focus on patterns is one way in which psychodynamic psychopharmacologists attend to patients' past experiences. More generally, prescribers are interested in patients' experiences with caregiving, treatment, and medications in order to anticipate the patients' potential psychological resistances to treatment. Although every competent psychopharmacologist will inquire about patients' past responses to medications, the psychodynamic psychopharmacologist strives to *understand* patients' history with medications. Complicated reactions to medications may also be transmitted transgenerationally, so patients' familial history of treatment experiences should be explored as well.

Focus on Interpersonal Experiences

Although psychodynamic psychopharmacologists are not focused explicitly on improving patients' interpersonal relationships (unless that is what the patient explicitly hopes to achieve from pharmacotherapy), a focus on functioning (vs. a focus on symptoms) often means that treatment is measured in terms of improved functioning in social roles. Furthermore, an assessment of interpersonal relationships is key to understanding relational patterns that may replay in relation to pharmacotherapy (e.g., a patient who has a history of "authority issues" may be expected to manifest these issues in psychiatric treatment).

Emphasize the Therapeutic Relationship

In biomedically oriented psychopharmacology, medications are seen as the key mutative factor. In psychodynamic psychopharmacology, however, it is often not at all clear how much the medication is the reason the patient gets better and how much "the doctor is the drug" (Balint 1957), contributing to outcomes by his or her very nature (McKay et al. 2006) or through the therapeutic alliance. What is clear is that the quality of the pharmacotherapeutic relationship has a significant impact on treatment outcomes, which is, in many cases, more potent than the active drug (Krupnick et al. 1996). Given this understanding, prescribers practicing psychodynamic psychopharmacology carefully attend to the prescriber–patient relationship; encourage patients to express their concerns, misgivings, and upsets with the prescriber; and maintain a focus on forming a sound therapeutic alliance.

Explore Patients' Wishes, Dreams, and Fantasies

Unless patients convey their feelings about pharmacotherapy by reporting dreams about medications, dream work has little place in the pharmacotherapeutic relationship. However, understanding patients' fantasies about medications (including those expressed in dreams) can be helpful in a number of ways. Showing interest in patients' mental lives, wishes, and fantasies is helpful for the alliance because patients can see that the prescriber is interested in them as a person. Understanding patients' fantasies about what medications do, how they work, and the doctor's reasons for prescribing them can help prescribers target treatment to align with the patients' wishes while also illuminating fantasies that would lead patients to fear and resist treatment. Given that patients' wishes for treatment are often complex, multilayered, and potentially irrational, it serves both patients and prescribers to attempt to gain a fuller picture of the patients' wishes and not limit treatment to simple symptom reduction. This allows for the development of a more solid alliance in which the prescribers and patients are more consciously working together rather than at cross-purposes. Illuminating patients' wishes may also create space to grapple with wishes that are irrational from a medical standpoint and that may otherwise turn into problems in the alliance.

Ordinary Medical Psychotherapy

Psychodynamic psychopharmacology is not a traditional depth therapy in the way of psychodynamic psychotherapy or psychoanalysis, although the approaches do share features in common. Psychodynamic psychopharmacologists do not attempt to illuminate patients' unconscious conflicts in a general sense to help them resolve those conflicts and have better lives. Rather, they prescribe (or do not prescribe) medications in such a way that the medications have the greatest benefit for the patients. To accomplish this task, however, particularly when prescribing for treatment-refractory patients, prescribers must develop a deeper understanding of these patients that accounts for their conflicts and resistances regarding psychiatric treatment. Forming an overall diagnosis (Balint 1967) that includes an understanding of "how the patient wants to use treatment" necessitates inquiry into patients' unconscious, their relational patterns, and their wishes for and fantasies about treatment. To elucidate these aspects requires using basic psychotherapeutic skills. In addition, prescribers' efforts to understand patients more deeply and to respond to them as unique individuals tend to strengthen the alliance, which appears, in and of itself, to improve pharmacological treatment outcomes (Krupnick et al. 1996) and enhances the potency of the drug called "doctor" (Balint 1957). Furthermore, this affords prescribers the information necessary to understand *how* to prescribe medications in a way that will be least likely to trigger unnecessary resistance.

An empathic interest in the *person* of a patient can go a long way. However, regardless of the prescriber's nonauthoritarian, caring commitment, patients can bring disturbed prior relationships with authority, caregiving, health, or medications into psychiatric treatment in ways that interfere with effective care. Taking a respectful and caring approach to these patients and making rational appeals that they make better use of medications are often insufficient to help them contain attitudes that are deeply held and largely unconscious. In this case, it may be necessary to engage these resistances more directly.

Interpretation is arguably the primary task of the psychodynamic psychotherapist, with the goal of helping patients extend conscious awareness and control over previously unconscious aspects of the psyche. Raising patients' consciousness is not the job of psychodynamic psychopharmacologists; their primary task is to prescribe. However, to prescribe effectively, they may have to engage in interpretation. One potential risk of combining psychodynamics with psychopharmacology is that a greater understanding of patients' dynamics can also be used in ways that diminish their authority. When the understanding of the patients' vulnerabilities is used primarily to persuade them into a particular attitude or course of action (e.g., to take their medications), this may be more properly understood as manipulation (Bibring 1954; Nevins 1990) rather than interpretation. Such manipulation is perhaps unavoidably a part of the psychopharmacological interaction, but prescribers working within a psychodynamic frame should be aware of these paternalistic dynamics and their potential consequences. Manipulation, even if used to push patients into making healthy choices, can undermine the patients' authority and the therapeutic alliance.

Psychodynamic psychopharmacology can be seen as a form of "ordinary medical psychotherapy"—that is, a kind of "6-minute psychotherapy" (Balint 1969; Weinberg and Mintz 2018)—that can be practiced alongside any ordinary, brief, and episodic medical encounter. It attends to the person of the patient and incorporates psychodynamic attitudes and skills to deepen understanding of the patient's wishes for treatment, to find common ground with the patient, and to understand, from a psychological perspective, reasons that treatment resistance may make sense, thus strengthening the working alliance. Efforts to illuminate the story behind treatment resistance and to help patients come into a relationship with treatment that is relatively unclouded by unhelpful transferences and unconscious resistances are akin to the skills used by the most sought-after physicians of any specialty.

Key Points

- A psychodynamically informed perspective on prescribing recognizes that patients' early life experiences with caregiving shapes how they orient, sometimes unhelpfully, toward treatment.

- Patients bring ambivalence and complicated feelings into the pharmacotherapeutic relationship in ways that are often unconscious.

- The practice of psychodynamic psychopharmacology shapes the role of patient and prescriber, positioning them as coinvestigators.

- Psychodynamic psychopharmacology shares characteristics of a psychodynamic psychotherapeutic approach to create a kind of "ordinary medical psychotherapy" that can be practiced during routine pharmacotherapy.

References

Ainsworth MDS, Bell SM: Attachment, exploration, and separation: illustrated by the behavior of one-year-olds in a strange situation. Child Dev 41(1):49–67, 1970 5490680

Baker E, Fee J, Bovingdon L, et al: From taking to using medication: recovery-focused prescribing and medicines management. Adv Psychiatr Treat 19(1):2–10, 2013

Balint E: A study of the doctor-patient relationship using randomly selected cases. J Coll Gen Pract 13(2):163–173, 1967

Balint E: The possibilities of patient-centered medicine. J R Coll Gen Pract 17(82):269–276, 1969 5770926

Balint M: The Doctor and His Patient and the Illness. London, Pitman, 1957

Bartholomew K, Horowitz LM: Attachment styles among young adults: a test of a four-category model. J Pers Soc Psychol 61(2):226–244, 1991

Bennett JK, Fuertes JN, Keitel M, et al: The role of patient attachment and working alliance on patient adherence, satisfaction, and health-related quality of life in lupus treatment. Patient Educ Couns 85(1):53–59, 2011 20869188

Bibring E: Psychoanalysis and the dynamic psychotherapies. J Am Psychoanal Assoc 2:745–770, 1954

Blagys MD, Hilsenroth MJ: Distinctive features of short-term psychodynamic-interpersonal psychotherapy: a review of the comparative psychotherapy process literature. Clin Psychol Sci Pract 7(2):167–188, 2000

Bowlby J: The nature of the child's tie to his mother. Int J Psychoanal 39(5):350–373, 1958 13610508

Bowlby J: Attachment and Loss, Vol 2: Separation, Anxiety and Anger. London, Hogarth, 1973

Ciechanowski PS, Katon WJ, Russo JE, et al: The patient-provider relationship: attachment theory and adherence to treatment in diabetes. Am J Psychiatry 158(1):29–35, 2001 11136630

Ciechanowski PS, Russo JE, Katon WJ, et al: Influence of patient attachment style on self-care and outcomes in diabetes. Psychosom Med 66(5):720–728, 2004 15385697

Clever SL, Ford DE, Rubenstein LV, et al: Primary care patients' involvement in decision-making is associated with improvement in depression. Med Care 44(5):398–405, 2006 16641657

Comninos AG, Grenyer BFS: The influence of interpersonal factors on the speed of recovery from major depression. Psychother Res 17(2):230–239, 2007

Cooper AM: Will neurobiology influence psychoanalysis? Am J Psychiatry 142(12):1395–1402, 1985 4073300

Frank JD: Eleventh Emil A. Gutheil memorial conference: therapeutic factors in psychotherapy. Am J Psychother 25(3):350–361, 1971 4936109

Freud S: The question of lay analysis (1926), in Standard Edition of the Complete Psychological Works of Sigmund Freud, Vol 20. Translated and edited by Strachey J. London, Hogarth, 1959, pp 177–258

Freud S: An outline of psycho-analysis (1940[1938]), in Standard Edition of the Complete Psychological Works of Sigmund Freud, Vol 23. Translated and edited by Strachey J. London, Hogarth, 1964, pp 139–207

Greenwald AG, Banaji MR: Implicit social cognition: attitudes, self-esteem, and stereotypes. Psychol Rev 102(1):4–27, 1995 7878162

Gutheil TG, Havens LL: The therapeutic alliance: contemporary meanings and confusions. Int J Psychoanal 6(4):467–481, 1979

Jensen KB, Kaptchuk TJ, Kirsch I, et al: Nonconscious activation of placebo and nocebo pain responses. Proc Natl Acad Sci USA 109(39):15959–15964, 2012 23019380

Krupnick JL, Sotsky SM, Simmens S, et al: The role of the therapeutic alliance in psychotherapy and pharmacotherapy outcome: findings in the National Institute of Mental Health Treatment of Depression Collaborative Research Program. J Consult Clin Psychol 64(3):532–539, 1996 8698947

McKay KM, Imel ZE, Wampold BE: Psychiatrist effects in the psychopharmacological treatment of depression. J Affect Disord 92(2–3):287–290, 2006 16503356

Nevins DB: Psychoanalytic perspectives on the use of medication for mental illness. Bull Menninger Clin 54(3):323–339, 1990 2207466

Parsons T: Illness and the role of the physician: a sociological perspective. Am J Orthopsychiatry 21(3):452–460, 1951 14857123

Sable P: What is adult attachment? Clin Social Work J 36(1):21–30, 2008

Shapiro ER: Finding a Place to Stand: Developing Self-Reflective Institutions, Leaders and Citizens. Manila, Philippines, Phoenix Publishing House, 2019

Simmel E: The psychoanalytic sanitarium and the psychoanalytic movement. Bull Menninger Clin 1(5):133–143, 1937

Tutter A: Medication as object. J Am Psychoanal Assoc 54(3):781–804, 2006 17009655

Tyrrell CL, Dozier M, Teague GB, et al: Effective treatment relationships for persons with serious psychiatric disorders: the importance of attachment states of mind. J Consult Clin Psychol 67(5):725–733, 1999 10535239

Waldinger RJ, Frank AF: Clinicians' experiences in combining medication and psychotherapy in the treatment of borderline patients. Hosp Community Psychiatry 40(7):712–718, 1989 2777227

Weinberg E, Mintz D: The overall diagnosis: psychodynamic psychiatry, six-minute psychotherapy, and patient-centered care. Psychiatr Clin North Am 41(2):263–275, 2018 29739525

• PART II •

Understanding Pharmacological Treatment Resistance

• CHAPTER 4 •

Psychodynamics of Pharmacological Treatment Resistance

Very shortly, you will be going onto your assigned wards. Within those wards, you will see over fifty of the sickest, craziest, most bizarre people you will ever encounter. They will be hallucinating, gesticulating, and delusional in the most grotesque ways. Every cell in your body will rebel and want to block out the experience. But here is the thing you must remember. Every one of those symptoms, as strange as they may seem to you, makes perfect sense to those people. Every single one has been evolved and carefully crafted, to try to deal with some impossible family situation. Every one represents an attempt by that person to adapt to the hand that fate has dealt him. You are to regard each one as an artistic, creative endeavor, to survive. Your job, and your only job, is to appreciate, and admire that effort!

—Elvin Semrad, M.D., addressing his first-year
psychiatric residents, circa 1968

Understanding Treatment Resistance

When patients are resistant to treatment, most treatment algorithms recommend ensuring first that the medical trials have been of adequate dosage and duration. When trials within a specific drug class have failed, common algorithms suggest prescribing medications with a different mechanism. If those strategies do not succeed, other types of treatments are recommended (e.g., electroconvulsive therapy, psychotherapy). At some point, prescribers must also consider whether the diagnosis is correct. These strategies are summed up in the five Ds (Csernansky and Hollister 1986):

• **D**iagnosis
• **D**osage

55

Table 4–1.   The six Ds of treatment resistance

Diagnosis
Dose
Duration of treatment
Putative mechanism of the **D**rug
Apply a **D**ifferent treatment
Dynamics

Source.   Adapted from Csernansky and Hollister 1986.

- **D**uration of treatment
- The putative mechanism of the **D**rug
- Use of a **D**ifferent treatment

Although some algorithms (e.g., Chehil et al. 2001) do recognize that psychosocial factors (e.g., character pathology, nonadherence, and other complicating and confounding factors) may contribute to treatment resistance, the recommended course of action to "manage accordingly" likely leaves many prescribers wanting. This gap is what psychodynamic psychopharmacology aims to address: how does one manage such complicating factors accordingly?

The first task in addressing psychosocial interferences with pharmacological treatment is to understand how and why these factors are interfering with the optimal use of medications. In other words, a thorough and complete analysis of pharmacotherapeutic treatment resistance adds a sixth D to Csernansky and Hollister's (1986) strategic approach: **D**ynamics (Table 4–1). Given the profound effects of psychosocial factors on medication response and the ubiquity of ambivalence about various aspects of treatment (e.g., issues of power and control, worries about the negative effects of medications, worries about stigma), any comprehensive approach to psychopharmacotherapy necessitates attention to these factors.

When patients' treatment resistance arises from the level of meaning, it is unlikely that primarily biomedical approaches to that resistance (e.g., using sub- or supratherapeutic dosages, trying second- and third-line treatments) will produce significantly better outcomes. Medication trials will fail repeatedly if patients fail to adhere to the prescribed regimen or repeatedly develop intolerable side effects, no matter the dosage or medication. Even if patients take their medications as prescribed, ambivalent feelings are likely to interfere with healthy outcomes (Mintz and Flynn 2012).

Dr. A, a 43-year-old woman who is currently supporting herself on alimony from a divorce 5 years prior, presents with major depression with anxious distress that started a few years before she separated from her husband, an upper-level pharmaceutical executive. Dr. A describes herself as having multiple chemical sensitivities that began with sensitivities to medications but now extend to other chemical substances (e.g., cleaning products, secondhand smoke). Preoccupied with her physical well-being, she takes a number of vitamins and nutraceutical treatments and can tolerate them without experiencing adverse consequences. However, she has failed multiple trials of selective serotonin reuptake inhibitors and serotonin-norepinephrine reuptake inhibitors because of the repeated emergence of intolerable side effects. She has also failed a few other trials, including tricyclic antidepressants as well as several medications she was prescribed for medical conditions. Her prescriber, recognizing that Dr. A's sensitivity to medications is likely to interfere with further trials, adopts a start-low, go-slow strategy, beginning bupropion at a dosage of 12.5 mg/day, which is less than one-tenth of a normal starting dosage. Even at this dosage, however, Dr. A develops both headaches and nausea that necessitate treatment discontinuation.

The prescriber realizes that further treatment is unlikely to be successful and seeks consultation with a nationally recognized psychopharmacologist who recognizes that the trouble is likely not a problem of actual chemical hypersensitivity but rather a problem of the meaning of the substances. Assuming that the patient is anxious about being harmed and is thus hyperalert to distressing somatic sensations, the psychopharmacologist recommends negotiating a placebo trial. Dr. A will begin receiving, with her consent, a placebo pill. At some point, however, that placebo will be replaced with active drug in the capsule, although the patient will not know when this change occurs. The dosage will thereafter gradually be escalated to a therapeutic level, again without the patient's awareness. The idea is to attempt to bypass her hyperattention to bodily states and her expectation of negative effects related to new medication and dosage increases. Although this is indeed a very clever solution, Dr. A (or her unconscious) is cleverer still, because she suddenly develops what she experiences as an allergy to the methylcellulose in the placebo capsule.

Patients who are hyperalert to being harmed and are prone to side effects (nocebo effects) are not an anomaly in clinical practice. They can easily stymie prescribers who are operating from a predominantly biomedical framework. Lowering dosages or prescribing medications with different or fewer side effects does not effectively address the problem because these patients are perfectly capable of producing their own side effects. The case of Dr. A demonstrates clearly that when treatment resistance arises from the level of meaning, it will likely only be addressed effectively at that level. This requires, first and foremost, a comprehensive diagnosis that includes an informed hypothesis of how and why dynamic factors are interfering with the patients' ability to use medications in a healthy way.

Psychodynamic Formulation of Pharmacological Treatment Resistance

Michael Balint (1957), in his classic work *The Doctor, His Patient and the Illness*, recommended developing a psychodynamic understanding of the origins of treatment resistance. What he referred to as an "overall diagnosis," or psychodynamic formulation, may guide prescribers in engaging patients' treatment resistance at the level of meaning, addressing the factors that interfere with treatment and optimizing the factors that are concordant with optimal outcomes. According to Enid Balint (1969), an effective dynamic understanding focuses not so much on patients' structural or psychological deficits as on the adaptive effort underlying their resistance: "These criteria cannot be in terms of such clichés as oral dependence, castrating mothers, immature egos, sexual inadequacy, and so on, or what really amounts to 'illness-centred medicine.'...The question is more one of how the patient wants to use the doctor" (p. 274). This is sound advice because it positions prescribers to respond empathically to treatment-resistant patients who might otherwise be experienced as difficult or even as simply hateful (Groves 1978) and helps them form an understanding around which an alliance may be formed.

There are as many different kinds of treatment resistance as there are treatment-resistant patients. Nevertheless, when formulating the dynamics of a patient's treatment resistance, it may be useful to consider that resistance as falling into broad categories. Some writers have suggested dynamic approaches to pharmacological treatment resistance that are based on character structure (Forrest 2004; Marcus 1990), but this approach tends toward an illness-centered understanding of the problem. Psychodynamic psychopharmacology posits that it is useful to consider the meaning and function of patients' treatment resistance because this approach lends itself more to an understanding of how to address that resistance. Groves (1978), for example, in his classic paper "Taking Care of the Hateful Patient," recognized that dynamic conflicts (e.g., around dependency) are often at the heart of complicated treatments in which patients not only resist treatment but also evoke strong negative feelings in the doctor. He suggested that once the dynamic origin of the patients' treatment resistance is identified, doctors are better able to respond empathically in ways that do not exacerbate a countertherapeutic dynamic.

Treatment resistance may also be thought of as falling into two broad (although not mutually exclusive) categories: patients who are treatment resistant *to* medications and those who are treatment resistant *from* medications (Table 4–2). Patients who are resistant *to* medications cannot allow a

Table 4–2. Manifestations of pharmacological treatment resistance

Treatment resistance *to* medications	Treatment resistance *from* medications
Ambivalence about treatment is prominent	Patient desires medications and reports they are effective
Ambivalence may not be conscious	Medications are turned to serve countertherapeutic ends
Ambivalence about	
Medication	Manifests in
Illness	Patient reports medications are helpful
Treaters	Often wants more medication
Manifests in	Functioning does not appear to improve
Nonresponse	Chronification
Nonadherence	Countertransference
Side effects interrupting treatment	Vague guilt or shame
Countertransference	
Frustration	
Helplessness	

medication to have its desired effect. Resistance in this category often takes the form of noncompliance with treatment. However, this category also includes a subgroup of patients who develop adverse psychological or physical responses to medications that are experienced as new or worsening symptoms or side effects and those who simply, albeit unconsciously, resist the treatment or its effects. On the other hand, patients who are resistant *from* medications generally present in quite the opposite way. They typically desire medications and often describe the medications as helpful. Although these patients feel helped, they do not seem to get better. In this case, it is not that medications are resisted but, rather, that the medications or the meanings attached to them are serving some countertherapeutic end. The treatment itself in some way adversely affects the patients' health. Although in such cases it would seem that medication discontinuation would be a reasonable approach, the patients are then also deprived of the potential benefits of the medication. Given that, in many cases, such harm from medications is moderated by meaning, treatment resistance from medications may often be addressed by illuminating the nature of the treatment resistance.

The dynamics of treatment resistance to and from medications are not mutually exclusive. In accordance with the principle of multiple functions (Waelder 1936/2007), a symptom, pathological attachment to medications, or treatment-interfering behavior such as nonadherence may simultaneously serve multiple functions. A patient may resist medications because she believes the medication stigmatizes her, while simultaneously internalizing the stigma attached to medications. As a consequence, she may view herself as hopelessly damaged, ultimately worsening her self-esteem and depression. This patient resists the treatment actively but still experiences iatrogenic effects attached to the medication, worsening her treatment resistance. Where treatment resistance is particularly recalcitrant, it is worth considering that the resistance may be serving multiple functions for the patient.

Key Points

- Psychodynamic sources of resistance to the healthy use of medications should be considered in cases of pharmacological treatment resistance.

- Treatment resistance may emerge either *to* medications, when patients are driven unconsciously to resist the medications, or *from* medications, when patients turn medications or their meanings to countertherapeutic ends.

- A psychodynamic formulation that considers patients' manifest and latent wishes for and fears of treatment can help guide their treatment.

References

Balint E: The possibilities of patient-centered medicine. J R Coll Gen Pract 17(82):269–276, 1969 5770926

Balint M: The Doctor and His Patient and the Illness. London, Pitman Medical, 1957

Chehil S, Devarajan S, Dursun SM: Pharmacologic management of refractory depression. Can Fam Physician 47:50–52, 2001 11212433

Csernansky JG, Hollister LE: Medical-management of refractory endogenous depressions. Hosp Formul 21(2):206, 1986

Forrest DV: Elements of dynamics II: psychodynamic prescribing. J Am Acad Psychoanal Dyn Psychiatry 32(2):359–380, 2004 15274501

Groves JE: Taking care of the hateful patient. N Engl J Med 298(16):883–887, 1978 634331

Marcus ER: Integrating psychopharmacotherapy, psychotherapy, and mental structure in the treatment of patients with personality disorders and depression. Psychiatr Clin North Am 13(2):255–263, 1990 2191280

Mintz DL, Flynn DF: How (not what) to prescribe: nonpharmacologic aspects of psychopharmacology. Psychiatr Clin North Am 35(1):143–163, 2012 22370496

Waelder R: The principle of multiple function: observations on over-determination. 1936. Psychoanal Q 76(1):75–92, discussion 93–117, 119–148, 2007 17294824

CHAPTER 5

Treatment Resistance to Medications

To array a man's will against his sickness is the supreme art of medicine.

—Henry Ward Beecher

Generally, patients have many reasons to resist the medications we prescribe. Patients are often quite ambivalent about their pharmacological care. That ambivalence may be about the medications themselves but may also represent ambivalence about the doctor (Waldinger and Frank 1989) or even about the illness (Table 5–1).

Ambivalence About Medications

Although Sir William Osler observed that "the desire to take medicine is perhaps the greatest feature which distinguishes man from animals" (Cushing 1925, p. 342), the desire to take medications is almost always melded with a desire to *not* take medications (or to not need medications). On the simplest level, the task of taking medications is a burden patients most likely would rather not have. Furthermore, the direct physical effects of medications are not always (or entirely) salubrious. Side effects may be anticipated and reacted to even when they do not occur. As noted in Chapter 2, expectations of harm from medications are quite common among patients, frequently even outweighing their expectations of being helped (Piguet et al. 2007).

Medications also carry noxious meanings as symbols of illness or deficit. Patients may experience their medications as a constant reminder that they are ill, and they sometimes operate under the fantasy that they can rid themselves of an illness by ridding themselves of the medication. This ambivalence is likely deepened further when others perceive the medications as a reminder of the patients' illness. When the meanings that others attach to pa-

Table 5–1.   Common sources of ambivalence about pharmacological treatment

Ambivalence about medications	Ambivalence about treaters	Ambivalence about illness
Medications cause physical harm (i.e., side effects)	Caregivers are unreliable	Symptoms are themselves gratifying (e.g., mania)
Medications are an imposition	Caregivers are out to meet their own needs	Symptoms provide practical compensation (e.g., disability)
Medications are a reminder of defect or deficit	Caregivers are harmful	Symptoms relieve patients of onerous responsibilities
Medications are stigmatizing	Caregivers are rejecting	Symptoms evoke caregiving
Medications represent dependency	Caregivers are paternalistic or controlling	Symptoms give patients power over others
Medications represent control by the doctor	Caregivers treat patients like symptoms	Symptoms serve defensive functions
Medications represent toxic or sexual intrusion		Symptoms express anger toward self or others
Medications disrupt equilibrium		Symptoms communicate what cannot be verbalized
		Symptoms represent rebellion against objectification

tients' medications are stigmatizing, those medications become more shameful, and medication adherence suffers (Sirey et al. 2001).

> Mr. B, a 20-year-old man, presents with a history of difficulty with social adjustment, mood reactivity, occasional aggressive outbursts, and almost daily cannabis use. He describes a tense and conflictual relationship with his divorced parents, who had a very conflictual marriage. In childhood, Mr. B was diagnosed with oppositional defiant disorder and major depressive disorder. From early adolescence, he has been prescribed several different selective serotonin reuptake inhibitors (SSRIs) and has worked with several psychiatric prescribers. Antidepressants appeared to partially stabilize and support his mood, but he is still dysphoric at his medicated baseline. He has made two suicide attempts, both in the context of conflict with a parent and during periods of nonadherence to prescribed medications. Mr. B's most recent attempt involved a small overdose of six to eight tablets of the antidepressant that he had not been taking after dropping out of treatment. He was briefly hospitalized and has been referred to the new prescriber.

At the time of this first meeting, Mr. B is living at home with his mother, 1 week after his most recent overdose. There is a great deal of tension between him and his mother. The psychiatrist inquires why he has not been taking the medications prescribed for him since his brief inpatient stay. "It just proves her right," the young man retorts. As they discuss the meaning of his statement, it becomes apparent that medications are used in the family in a stigmatizing and defensive way. Whenever he and his mother argue, for example, his mother asks, "Have you taken your meds?" In this defensive arrangement, medications have come to mean that he is crazy, that the areas of disagreement with his mother are simply pathological, and that his objections to her behavior (or even provocations) are distortions, mere signs of mental illness. Taking medications has become disempowering and stigmatizing and thus unbearable. Mr. B's unconscious reasoning is that if he does not take medications, he will not be vulnerable to such projections, leading him to refuse potentially helpful treatment.

In manifold ways, the pharmacological effect of a medication and its meaning may come into opposition, mobilizing patients' ambivalence. Areas of ambivalence from patients' relational lives are often echoed powerfully in their relationships with medications. Patients who are easily narcissistically wounded often experience medications as a narcissistic injury. Patients who react strongly to feeling controlled in relationships likely also worry about ways that medications represent a form of control. A patient who is concerned about "being turned into a zombie" by medications may be worried not only about being transformed into the living dead but also about falling under the control of a zombie master—a psychopharmacologist, according to the original zombie mythology. Patients who are conflicted, both dependent and fearful of dependency, may want to stop medications that are particularly helpful because of increased fears that their need for the medication or dependence on the prescriber will render them vulnerable.

Ms. C, a 26-year-old woman, seeks treatment for paralysis in her romantic and professional lives. Both her relationships and her jobs tend to last no longer than a few weeks or months. Her employment is often interrupted by symptoms of chronic, low-grade depression, when she feels simply too depressed, physically unwell, and unmotivated to get out of bed. Between jobs, she spends her days perusing the internet and social media and smoking cannabis. At her pharmacotherapy intake, she endorses symptoms consistent with persistent depressive disorder and moderate cannabis use disorder. Although she has a history of sexual abuse by a teacher in middle school, she denies any symptoms of PTSD. She failed to respond to multiple prior antidepressant trials but admits that, like her employment and relationships, her antidepressant trials generally ended within a few weeks. On further exploration, it appears that nonadherence frequently interrupts treatments when Ms. C seems to be emerging from depression and concludes that she does not need antidepressants. However, when she does not find a medication effective, she tends to stay on it for a longer period of time. When Dr. X asks her about this, Ms. C speaks of her hope that the medication might someday change and become effective.

Ms. C describes her early life as characterized by emotional neglect, with highly career-focused parents who worked long hours. She believes that she was partially responsible for her abuse in middle school because she was herself desperately looking for attention from her teacher as a replacement for the attention she was missing at home. Although she does not exhibit classic symptoms of PTSD, Ms. C is aware that she feels highly conflicted about her emotional needs, especially in relation to others. She hypothesizes that she may destroy romantic relationships when feelings of dependency emerge either in herself or in her partner, evoking her contempt. Her pharmacotherapist, Dr. X, suggests that because her dependency made her vulnerable to being traumatized as a child, she not only destroys interpersonal relationships when dependency emerges but also seems to stop medications when she begins to feel dependent. Although she is unsure whether this feels true to her experience, Ms. C is able to observe that she is more able to adhere to medications when she does not believe they are effective.

Patients who have been traumatized, particularly if that trauma is being processed preverbally, in the body and in action, may be inclined to act out some aspect of that trauma around medications. Ingesting medications is one concrete area in which the patient's body is acted upon by the doctor and in which the doctor may be experienced as putting something harmful into the patient's body. When patients experience medications as echoing some aspect of a past trauma, they understandably experience ambivalence about treatment, although that ambivalence may not be conscious. Prescribers for such patients commonly experience a dilemma because they are inevitably pulled in to reenact some aspect of the trauma that the patient has not yet put into words. By prescribing medication, they may believe that they are being invited into the role of abuser, but if they do not prescribe medication they then become identified with the parent who does nothing to interrupt the patient's suffering or abuse.

Ms. D is a 23-year-old woman from an affluent professional family. Anxious as a child, she now presents with a range of symptoms, including dissociation with significant loss of time, nightmares, flashbacks of previous trauma, and avoidance of almost anything that she might find arousing. She scratches, cuts, and burns herself on a regular basis. She is passively but not actively suicidal. Ms. D also experiences auditory hallucinations of degrading voices and tactile sensations of sexual molestation. Although her parents are emphatic that she needs treatment for a psychotic illness, she has herself recently begun to recount a narrative of abuse by her father, a physician with an alcohol use disorder. This is complicated for her because she experiences her father, in many ways, as the better of the two parents. Whereas he has always been caring and supportive, her mother has always seemed cold, critical, and rejecting. To make matters more complicated, Ms. D reports that the abuse was closely connected with caregiving. Whenever she went to her father for caregiving, she was likely to be forced (or pulled, she could not tell) into sexual acts; emotional support turned into caresses that seemed benign at first but became overtly sexual, culminating on some occasions in her performing oral sex on her father.

Ms. D previously tried several different serotonergic antidepressants and antipsychotics but was sensitive to side effects, including dyspepsia, sedation, worsening nightmares, and a range of paradoxical reactions, including worsening anxiety and increased self-harm in dissociated states. Considering how the doctor–patient relationships potentially echoed aspects of her relationship with her father, it is not surprising that her relationship with medication has proven to be so complicated. Both with her physician father and her prescribing psychiatrist, there is an explicit offer of comfort that is manifestly caring, but in both cases the scenario ends with the patient putting something into her mouth that makes her sick. Her prescriber initiates several brief trials of SSRIs and GABAergic medications but discontinues these trials very quickly when Ms. D reports the emergence of side effects.

As depicted in these vignettes, patients who are vulnerable to feelings of powerlessness are often particularly prone to feeling disrupted by medication effects. Furthermore, as noted in Chapter 2, members of socially disadvantaged groups are especially likely to have medication trials interrupted by the emergence of nocebo effects. Similarly, patients who are characterologically acquiescent are prone to interpret bodily sensations associated with medications as harmful. It is as though these patients, who feel unable to say "no" straightforwardly in words, instead say it with their bodies.

When patients have a tenuous sense of self, changes in their experience of their body or mind may catastrophically disrupt their sense of stability or equilibrium. For example, a patient with significant psychotic liabilities may find medication effects to be destabilizing not only because of their undesirable effects on his psychotic defenses but also because of disruptions to his body ego. When beset by shifting phantasmagorical realities, sometimes the only thing patients can count on is how it feels, concretely, to be in their own body. When medications introduce subtle shifts in interoceptive feedback (e.g., changes in tension or fatigue in the body), these patients may come to believe that medications introduce too great a disruption in the bedrock of their perception of reality, increasing psychotic anxiety or being experienced as a dangerous threat to the self. This can lead to nonadherence (if the patient is able to resist the doctor's prescription). Alternately, changes in a patient's body ego can produce mounting nocebo responses or anxiety-driven psychotic elaboration of symptoms (if the patient cannot resist the doctor and believes that he or she must acquiesce to the prescription). For example, in order to deny or contain his psychotic anxieties as a danger to or within the self, the patient elaborates and focuses on a concrete problem that becomes the source of anxiety, such as a belief that a medication has caused his penis to shrink.

Patients with a false-self organization (Winnicott 1955), or as-if personality (Deutsch 1942/2007), may also be prone to disruption in sense of self related to medication effects. These patients have deeply buried their more authentic feelings and identity to shape themselves to the desires of others, resulting in a very tenuous sense of self. They cannot often tell what is theirs and what they have adopted from others in order to be pleasing. In the same vein, they may find that psychic changes introduced by medications create significant confusion about what is them and what is the medication.

> Ms. E, a superficially high-functioning medical student, presents for treatment of depression and significant weight loss from somatized gastric pain. Her habitual efforts at attempting to become what others wanted her to be has left her feeling empty, with almost no sense of agency. One of her medications promotes weight loss, but the alternatives would likely promote weight gain. Her psychiatrist-psychotherapist, believing that his first duty is to "do no harm," wants to change the medication to avoid colluding with further weight loss, but Ms. E objects. When the doctor explores the patient's resistance, with the hope that they can both gain insight into how her resistance or reaction may connect to her broader life struggles, it becomes clear that Ms. E experiences the possibility of a medication effect as a threat to her identity. Specifically, while working in her therapy to find a more authentic experience of herself, she fears that if she gains weight, she will not know whether this is a consequence of her effort to care for herself better or is a function of the medication.

Ambivalence About Illness

Although they want to be rid of their illness, patients may consciously or unconsciously also value it. This can easily contribute to treatment resistance. On the most concrete level, symptoms such as mania can be immediately gratifying, leading patients to resist treatments that would undo these gratifications. Illnesses often provide patients with secondary gains, such as the opportunity to be treated in the sick role, escape onerous responsibilities, or receive other concrete benefits. Paradoxically, patients whose personal histories have involved extensive experiences of disempowerment may easily find that their infirmities have given them a kind of power that they never had when well. Such patients are likely to struggle with forces in themselves that run counter to the intent of treatment, leading to behaviors and attitudes that interfere with an optimal response to pharmacotherapy.

Patients may also become attached to symptoms when those symptoms serve important defensive functions. Symptoms may help patients manage intolerable affects, such as when a patient cultivates feelings of grandiosity to blind herself to feelings related to vulnerability or loss. As such, when trying to understand the nature of psychiatric treatment resistance, it is often helpful to look for ways that symptoms serve subtle defensive functions.

> Ms. F, an unmarried woman in her early 50s, presents for residential treatment of treatment-refractory psychosis. Although she has a 30-year history of schizophrenia, her symptoms have worsened over the past decade despite multiple medication trials. She is admitted on a typical neuroleptic but continues to experience frequent hallucinations and delusions. In addition, she is quite socially isolated, rarely interacting with people other than her aging parents. Although a newer atypical neuroleptic is clearly warranted, Ms. F is profoundly resistant to this idea because she is convinced that if she tries one of these medications, she will become depressed and kill herself. She is so concerned about this that whenever her psychiatric prescriber introduces a new medication, she becomes unmanageably anxious and her psychotic symptoms immediately escalate, further convincing her that the medications are a threat. Usually within a few days, her doctor concludes that the new medications exacerbate her condition and returns her to her previous regimen.
>
> Prior to entering treatment, Ms. F was living in her parents' home. Her parents' concern that they are aging and will soon be unable to support her is one of the manifest reasons Ms. F began residential treatment. She has lived with her parents since her mid-20s, when she became pregnant and gave birth to a son. Despite some psychotic symptoms, she competently raised him with her parents' help. Ms. F's psychosis seemed to worsen, however, after her son succumbed to brain cancer at the age of 5 years.
>
> Over time, the unconscious logic of Ms. F's treatment resistance becomes more apparent. Her hallucinations consist largely of hearing the voice of her child, which serves to interrupt her profound loneliness. Furthermore, among Ms. F's most common delusions is a conviction that she not only has the power to cure deadly diseases but also holds the secret for raising the dead. To lose these symptoms is thus tantamount to losing her child, who is being kept alive through her psychotic restitution (Deutsch 1938; Nevins 1977). Understandably, Ms. F experiences medications as a threat. Furthermore, her seemingly delusional belief that atypical neuroleptics will make her suicidally depressed is subjectively true. If these medications work, her child will be gone, and her grief could overwhelm her already limited capacities, leading her to suicidal despair.

Patients may become unconsciously attached to symptoms when those symptoms come to express something that cannot otherwise be communicated with words. The suffering inflicted by symptoms makes them a particularly well-suited vehicle for enacting hateful or aggressive impulses. To the extent that symptoms hurt and frustrate others close to the patient (e.g., doctors, family members, and other caregivers), they can effectively communicate the patient's unspoken anger. This communication may even be more powerful and effective when directed at the prescriber, who feels not only distress at the patient's suffering but also helpless, inadequate, or even guilty. The opportunity to communicate inexpressible anger often is secretly more gratifying than the opportunity to be rid of symptoms, resulting in various clandestine efforts to defeat the action of medications.

Patients can also ambivalently defeat medications when their symptoms serve to express anger directed not outwardly but inwardly, toward the self. When patients are struggling with deep-seated guilt or using suffering to punish unwanted yearnings, masochistic gratifications may outweigh the potential gratifications from symptom reduction, at least unconsciously. Pharmacological treatment of such patients may benefit from psychotherapeutic work to help them learn healthier ways to channel aggression. In contrast, symptoms may also enact patients' love and feelings of dependency that they do not otherwise know how to navigate. The prospect of being relieved of symptoms can be quite alarming, particularly when the patients' relationship with their mental health professional provides more caring attention than they have ever experienced or imagined.

> Ms. G is a chronically downtrodden woman in her early 40s who has been in treatment for generalized anxiety, panic, and depression since her teenage years. Her mother succumbed to substance use when Ms. G was young, and Ms. G lived with a number of extended family members before settling in with her paternal grandmother, who is now deceased. Ms. G has also been treated for bulimia (in her teens, now resolved), PTSD (from sexual abuse by an aunt's boyfriend), and cannabis abuse. She tends to live a small life, working infrequently and socializing mainly with extended family (cousins and nieces). She often uses alcohol to manage her anxiety when socializing with friends. She has had multiple therapists but has been with her current psychiatrist for 15 years. Pharmacotherapy (with a serotonergic antidepressant, GABAergic anticonvulsant, and atypical neuroleptic) has seemed helpful; her panic is well controlled, and her PTSD reactivity has faded into the background. More recently, she has been holding a part-time job.
>
> Ms. G's doctor suggests that the atypical neuroleptic she is taking may no longer be necessary. Although she offers some faint protest at first, she agrees that it is probably worth considering. They plan to discuss this further at their next appointment. Several weeks later, Ms. G requests an emergency appointment because her anxiety and depression have worsened, and she is unable to tolerate the stress of her job. Rather than reducing her medications, she requests more. The lack of a clear proximal stressor leads her doctor to conclude that the suggestion she might not need one of her medications is the likely stressor, and he hypothesizes that she has become alarmed that this suggestion is a prelude to abandonment. From this perspective, her worsening symptoms seem to be an unconscious effort to preserve a dependent connection to one of the more reliable caregivers in her life. She is unable to protest or to voice her dependent anxiety, so she acts it out instead through her decompensation.

Approaching such symptoms from a primarily biomedical perspective (e.g., more aggressive prescribing) leaves prescribers with limited tools for addressing this form of treatment resistance. Interventions to increase the efficacy of the medication regimen are counteracted by increasing efforts to remain ill and preserve the needed therapeutic relationship. This may be unconsciously recognized by systems of care or prescribers who establish treatment frames and develop prescriber–patient relationships that are noxious enough to prevent their patients from developing feelings of dependency.

Negative Transference: Ambivalence About Treaters

Patients who have primitive object relations experience others in stark ways that lack complexity and are related to developmentally early ways of experiencing. For example, someone who is disappointing would quickly come to be experienced as all bad and dangerous. Such patients are likely to bring this problem into the pharmacotherapeutic relationship. The ingestion of a pill may activate positive object representations, such as the oral gratification of the nursing situation for patients who have predominantly positive early experiences, but it may activate profoundly negative object representations in patients whose early experiences were unduly traumatic or neglectful. For example, for patients who have been sexually abused, the act of putting a pill into their mouths and swallowing it may activate toxic experiences of sexual intrusion or other forms of bodily control by another person, ultimately interfering with optimal use of medications. At times, patients recruit negative attitudes toward treaters as justification to resist treatments that threaten the elegant solutions that illness can provide. Such *transference resistances*, as Freud called them, likely must be addressed if these patients are to receive optimal benefit from psychopharmacological treatment.

Regardless of patients' ambivalence about illness and regardless of the doctor, many patients enter therapeutic relationships with preconceived biases against and negative reactions to caregivers. These transferences often derive from the patients' most basic lessons about caregiving, lessons that have colored the psychological filters through which they experience other caregiving relationships. If patients' early caregiving models were neglectful or self-preoccupied, they may often expect and experience self-centeredness in their caregivers, eroding the potential for trust and comfort. This, in turn, has adverse effects on the treatment alliance. Dismissive attachment is likely to emerge, especially when caregiving has been reliably neglectful, which has been shown to undercut health behaviors that promote better outcomes, including medication adherence (Ciechanowski et al. 2004). In a related situation, when caregivers have been hurtful or abusive, patients will have such expectations not only of medications but also relationally; when early caregivers have been rejecting, patients may experience treatments as suffused with rejection, if not representing rejection itself.

> Mr. H, a college-aged transgendered male patient, enters outpatient treatment for depression and anxiety. He complains particularly of chronic insomnia related to nightly panic attacks. Extensive medication trials have been repeatedly unsuccessful or intolerable. He comes from at least three generations of irritably obsessive people but is misattuned to his family, who have regarded him as cranky and demanding from infancy, projectively locating the family pathology in Mr. H as the one who is irritable and causes problems for others. Consequently, he believes his family is always trying to "stifle" him.
>
> Mr. H begins a trial of an SSRI for depression and panic. Soon after, he complains of "emotional deadness," a known side effect of this medication. Although the therapist-prescriber experiences him as less overwhelmed and more able to engage productively in self-exploration, Mr. H finds the experience intolerable and argues that he is too cut off from his emotions to use the psychotherapy. He requests to stop the medications and eventually does so. As treatment continues, the psychiatrist works with Mr. H to decipher the unconscious logic of this side effect. During and after the SSRI trial, Mr. H frequently responds in a self-critical way when he believes he has complained too much. For example, in the sessions, he finds himself irritably interjecting, "Oh, just put me in a cage and throw a blanket over me" or "Can't you just turn me into a zombie?" Although his doctor experiences these comments as an opportunity to better understand and work through Mr. H's anger, it becomes increasingly clear that Mr. H fears his emotionality has been intolerable to the doctor. As such, the success of the medication in quieting his anxiety makes the entire treatment feel like a rejection, echoing his view of his parents as "stifling." Based on this transference expectation, he experiences the SSRI as shutting him down and shutting him up, and intolerably so, because of the broader implications.

Patients' deepest and earliest suspicions about caregiving have also too frequently been reenacted and proven in their varied interactions with the mental health system. Indeed, as Fowler et al. (2011) noted, treatment resistance may emerge as patients' protest against a biomedically reductionistic system that would reduce them from a subject to a biological object, render their symptomatic world meaningless, and deauthorize them, thus making them dependent on their doctor for health. Their rejection of or rebellion against treatment is, in such cases, a refusal to be objectified within a biomedical system of meaning and may represent these patients' best efforts to assert the importance of their humanity.

When prescribers do not recognize deep yet often-hidden medical mistrust in patients, they may miss or otherwise be unprepared to address disguised negative transferences. When these patients are healthy enough to mobilize a straightforward resistance, they cannot submit trustfully to the medication because they experience it as harmful. Such patients are often recognizable by the recurrent struggles for control that occur around medications. They question prescribers' motivations, express fears of loss of control, show particular interest in the side effects of the medications (i.e., the prescribers' capacity to harm them), or will negotiate in excruciating detail the timing and dosages of the pills, raising the question of whether the prescribers should insist on the rational use of medications or tolerate patients' irrational efforts at control for some time-limited therapeutic purpose. If the prescriber asserts control, the patient may attempt to regain control of the medications by controlling the doctor. In this scenario, the patient no longer tells the doctor the relevant truth but instead presents a distorted symptom picture. This is coupled with urgent displays of affect intended to coerce the doctor into prescribing a medication regimen that the patient believes is within *his or her* control (Koenigsberg 1994). Patients who have resolved, consciously or unconsciously, to never again allow themselves to feel powerless may also project their disavowed powerlessness onto the prescriber in the form of projective identification.

> Ms. I, a 17-year-old biracial high school dropout, presents for treatment of a major depressive disorder with anxious distress because her primary care physician is no longer able to manage her depression. She has struggled with depression since at least the age of 15 years, when she first began to have difficulty in school. She left school and dropped out of many extracurricular activities, passively refusing to get out of bed or to leave the house for months at a time. This has created much distress in her perfectionistic, academically driven family. Although her family has tried multiple ways to motivate her, they have now backed off in a desperate and defeated paralysis after Ms. I attempted suicide by ingesting her mother's blood pressure medications following an argument.
>
> The psychiatrist immediately has an inkling that a powerfully controlling mother is likely somehow involved in the patient's troubles because he, too, is uncharacteristically filled with anxiety in the face of the mother's high expectations and challenging demand for results. No longer able comfortably to pressure her daughter, she brings all of her forceful anxiety to bear on the doctor, whom she expects to quickly get her daughter back on her trajectory to success. Although the doctor identifies with the patient, he succumbs to the mother's demand, which he then passes on to the patient as an unusually zealous effort to help her. Ms. I, however, will no longer allow herself to feel powerless. Although she accepts a prescription, she supplants the doctor, rejecting his directions and taking the medication according to her whim, first taking less than prescribed, then quickly escalating the dosage beyond what is recommended, and then taking less again after she develops side effects. This is repeated through several medication trials, while she fails to improve substantially. Caught between the patient and her mother, the doctor feels in-

creasingly helpless and controlled, now forced to feel those feelings that the patient is unwilling to bear.

When patients resist treatment, either actively or passively, prescribers often experience aversive countertransference reactions, such as frustration and anger or helplessness and resigned detachment. Indeed, a range of responses is normal and arguably crucial to understanding the patients' trouble. In fact, such countertransference may be the first clue that psychological dynamics of resistance to treatment are at play, aiding prescribers in developing a comprehensive formulation. Furthermore, recognizing that countertransference reactions provide valuable information may help prescribers to not be so buffeted by their own emotional reactions, preserving some equanimity. Seldom when prescribers act out countertransference does it promote a positive response to treatment. More likely, the failure of empathy will serve to reinforce dynamics that promote treatment resistance.

Key Points

- Treatment resistance *to* medications may be rooted in patients' ambivalence toward medications, a common phenomenon that is known adversely to affect medication outcomes.

- Unconscious (and conscious) secondary gains arouse ambivalence about illness, turning patients unconsciously against treatment.

- Unconsciously held negative expectations of caregiving may position patients to be as much adversaries as allies in the pharmacotherapeutic relationship.

- Experiences of powerlessness are typically fertile grounds for negative reactions to treatment and medications and sources of negative transference.

References

Ciechanowski P, Russo J, Katon W, et al: Influence of patient attachment style on self-care and outcomes in diabetes. Psychosom Med 66(5):720–728, 2004 15385697
Cushing H: The Life of Sir William Osler. New York, Oxford University Press, 1925
Deutsch H: Folie a deux. Psychoanal Q 7(3):307–318, 1938
Deutsch H: Some forms of emotional disturbance and their relationship to schizophrenia. 1942. Psychoanal Q 76(2):325–344, discussion 345–386, 2007 17503622

Fowler JC, Plakun EM, Shapiro ER: Treatment resistance, in Treatment Resistance and Patient Authority: The Austen Riggs Reader. Edited by Plakun EM. New York, WW Norton, 2011, pp 6–23

Koenigsberg HW: The combination of psychotherapy and pharmacotherapy in the treatment of borderline patients. J Psychother Pract Res 3(2):93–107, 1994 22700184

Nevins DB: Adverse response to neuroleptics in schizophrenia. Int J Psychoanal Psychother 6:227–241, 1977 914437

Piguet V, Cedraschi C, Dumont P, et al: Patients' representations of antidepressants: a clue to nonadherence? Clin J Pain 23(8):669–675, 2007 17885345

Sirey JA, Bruce ML, Alexopoulos GS, et al: Perceived stigma as a predictor of treatment discontinuation in young and older outpatients with depression. Am J Psychiatry 158(3):479–481, 2001 11229992

Waldinger RJ, Frank AF: Transference and the vicissitudes of medication use by borderline patients. Psychiatry 52(4):416–427, 1989 2685859

Winnicott DW: Metapsychological and clinical aspects of regression within the psychoanalytical set-up. Int J Psychoanal 36(1):16–26, 1955 14353557

• CHAPTER 6 •

Treatment Resistance From Medications

The person who takes medicine must recover twice, once from the disease and once from the medicine.

—Sir William Osler, M.D., C.M.

Patients may also develop treatment resistance in relation to medications that they neither fear nor resist. These patients will often ask for medications and experience them as valuable and effective. The prescriber may observe that the medication produces a reduction in symptoms, yet the patient does not get better in terms of his or her overall psychosocial functioning. In fact, despite reported symptom reduction, the patient seems somehow to be getting worse or becoming chronically ill. In these situations, medications may actually be turned to serve countertherapeutic ends, either consciously or unconsciously. The countertransference in such patients is often one of unease, guilt, or shame. Although the patient reports that the medications are helpful and perhaps even demands more medications, the prescriber still believes something is wrong and may feel some vague sense of participating in something perverse or fear that the patient is gradually becoming chronically ill.

Medications may contribute directly to chronicity, such as when sedating medications rob patients of their energy and drive or worsen their cognition (Husa et al. 2017), resulting in impairment of overall functioning. In cases of straightforward iatrogenesis, appropriate strategies require directly addressing these symptoms at the biomedical level (e.g., changing medications, reducing dosages, adding other medications to counteract the iatrogenic effects). More often, however, it is not the direct biological effects of the medication that promote treatment resistance but, rather, the meanings ascribed or the defensive functions attached to the medications that interfere with patients' agency or overall adaptive capacity. In this situation, when

75

Table 6–1.   Common dynamics of treatment resistance from
              medications

Medications misused in explicitly countertherapeutic ways (e.g., self-harm,
  recreational use)
Medications contributing to negative identity
Medications deauthorizing patients
Medications deskilling patients
Medications used defensively to avoid self-awareness and responsibility
Medications used defensively to replace people
Medications used to avoid healthy developmental steps
Medication effects used to communicate experiences of harm
Medications and enactment

treatment resistance is a function of meaning, it is likely to be most helpful
for prescribers to address the problem at its origin.

Because treatment resistance from medications is seldom concrete and
obvious, such as when patients misuse their prescribed medications through
acts of self-harm or recreational use, prescribers may easily be unaware that
they have become a participant in the development of treatment resistance.
When this occurs, the prescriber often has unwittingly colluded with defensive structures in the patient that act counter to the overall intent of treatment. Recognizing treatment resistance from medications (Table 6–1) often
requires that prescribers hold a broad view of the aims of treatment. In other
words, treatment is not simply defined as the absence of symptoms but as a
measure of health, resilience, self-satisfaction, adaptability, and capacity to
work and love. Prescribers who focus more narrowly on symptomatic mea-
sures (e.g., symptom checklists) as indicators of treatment success are perhaps more likely to see only the modest success of the treatments in reducing
certain target symptoms while missing that the patient is actually becoming
less functional.

When Medications Support
a Negative Identity

Biological explanations attached to medications are one mechanism by
which patients may be harmed by medications, thus contributing to treatment resistance. A negative identity (Erikson 1959, 1968) may develop in the
context of pharmacotherapy when patients defensively identify with and
own unfavorable elements of a self-concept that become attached to medications. Patients with mild to moderate depression who see their illness pri-

marily through a biological lens tend to be more pessimistic, have a reduced sense of self-efficacy (Kemp et al. 2014), and obtain less benefit from antidepressant trials (Sullivan et al. 2003). When patients internalize negative self-attributions of defect, incompetence, or badness attached to medications (or to diagnoses), these can be incorporated into a pathogenic sense of the self that interferes with their recovery. These effects on identity may be especially profound in cases in which patients have been medicated since childhood and have not been afforded the opportunity to examine the impact of those medications on their identity. Such patients may be left with profound and distressing questions about who they really are and struggle to know what their natural capacities are as distinct from the capacities that are provided or supported by medications (Mintz 2019).

When Medications Serve Defensive Functions

Medications can also interfere with healthy coping and development when they function as inexact interpretations (Glover 1931; Nevins 1990) that bolster maladaptive defenses. An inexact interpretation delivered from a medical authority offers patients a plausible-enough explanation of their mind or behavior that they can utilize to explain away and effectively repress their distressing thoughts and feelings, such as those related to guilt and shame. Glover (1931) noted that general practitioners were particularly likely to play this role by suggesting that patients' psychic troubles are biological in nature and offering prescriptions for medications, rest, and so on. By offering such an explanation, "intuitively [the doctor] attempts to deal at once with the patient's superficial anxiety layers and his deepest guilt layers" (p. 410). Psychopharmacologists, operating from a biomedically reductionistic perspective, hold a similar role in contemporary practice. By using their authority to reduce patients' distress through developing and fortifying patients' defensive structures, Glover noted that psychopharmacologists are "in this respect the lineal descendant of the first magical pharmacologists" (p. 410).

> Ms. J, a 31-year-old recently divorced mother, presents for treatment of bipolar II disorder. She recently moved to be closer to her family after finalizing a contentious divorce. Both Ms. J and her ex-husband have documented histories of heavy alcohol use, violent conflict in the home, and neglect of their 6-year-old daughter. As a result, Ms. J's daughter has recently been removed from their care and is living with Ms. J's mother. Ms. J has been unemployed for several years and is seeking disability for her bipolar disorder. She is clear from the outset that she is nervous about meeting a new doctor because of her previous difficulties finding a psychopharmacologist who could accurately understand her trouble.

Although initially prescribed lamotrigine for bipolar disorder, Ms. J is now also taking a high-dosage GABAergic anticonvulsant three times a day for anxiety and mood stabilization, a high-dosage nightly atypical neuroleptic for mood stabilization and sleep, and a relatively low-dosage selective serotonin reuptake inhibitor (SSRI) for anxiety and bipolar depression. The dosages of her more sedating medications have been increased in the context of the dissolution of her marriage. Ms. J believes that her medications are "not quite right…but pretty good." She continues to experience some symptoms of bipolar disorder, including mood swings; irritability, leading to frequent arguments with family; racing thoughts; and impulsivity in multiple domains, including sex and spending. Her sleep is well controlled with her current medications but becomes disrupted when she does not take her sedating antipsychotic at night. Because of problems with her current medications, Ms. J reports that she episodically has to "self-medicate" with alcohol, although she recognizes that this is a bad way to approach her problems and believes she could easily abstain once her anxiety and mood swings have been effectively controlled.

During their first meeting, the psychiatrist works to better understand Ms. J's psychiatric symptoms. From the history provided, it is not clear if her mood lability is characterologically based or indeed caused by frank bipolarity. However, the moment her psychiatrist raises a question about the nature of her bipolarity, Ms. J's anxiety escalates dramatically. The psychiatrist's anxiety also escalates because Ms. J reacts as though the doctor has harmed her by simply raising the question. He fears a confrontation with the intense irritability she described. It seems that pushing the point would risk the therapeutic alliance, lumping the new psychiatrist in with the others who have failed to understand her. He considers whether it might be better to develop an alliance with Ms. J before raising more distressing questions.

Why does Ms. J have such a strong reaction to a question of her diagnosis? There are likely many reasons. On some level, this experience may represent her grief over losing her previous psychopharmacologist or a fear of falling under control of someone she does not trust. More pointedly, however, is that questions about her diagnosis likely threaten a potent defense. Patients who rely on primitive defenses (e.g., splitting) commonly ruin their lives and damage those they love and need through their volatile, chaotic, and defensive style of engagement. Struggling with overwhelming feelings of guilt, these patients mobilize splitting defenses further and seek to manage their sense of "badness" by locating it outside themselves, often in another person (e.g., "I only did that bad thing because you provoked it in me").

In this case, Ms. J received the medication with a diagnosis that served as an inexact interpretation that said, "Your bad behavior is not you; it is your disease." This dynamic supports a defensive splitting in the patient and a disavowal of agency. She now attributes her badness (e.g., impulsive or destructive behaviors) to illness, while the remaining goodness resides in herself, and she backs up this defense with medical authority. For Ms. J, the diagnosis is profound because it powerfully relieves her of painful guilt and self-hatred, and she feels immediately better. Her previous treater seemed to take her reports of improved mood as confirmation of the diagnosis and evidence of a therapeutic response to lamotrigine, although the previous psychopharmacologist could also have been tempted to collude with this defense because the decrease in Ms. J's excruciating self-hatred was so relieving to both of them. Unfortunately, the final result of such an inexact interpretation is that although the patient feels better, she does worse. Ms. J biologizes her troubles so that she no longer feels responsible for her destructive behaviors. Now that her "bad behaviors" are symptoms of bipolar disorder, they are no longer her problem but are the responsibility of her prescriber. Thus, she gives them free rein and, despite escalating dosages of medications that she experiences as helpful, her marriage has eroded to the point of breaking and her daughter has been removed from her custody.

When Medications Replace Healthy Capacities

Psychiatric patients often form complex and pathogenic relationships with their affective lives because feelings have seemed to fail to serve a useful purpose. In healthy development, affects can be understood to serve a "signal function" (Freud 1926/1959; Solbakken et al. 2011; Wong 1999). Neurobiologically, affective systems have developed over the course of human evolution to help individuals navigate the world and register salient aspects of their experiences. Negative affects insistently alert people to physical and emotional dangers. By virtue of their experience as positive or negative, affects also engage the motivational system, prompting people to change their behavior in some way to respond to the perceived threat or reward. Anxiety points to physical and social dangers in the world. Likewise, some feelings of guilt and shame can serve as behavioral reminders of how to effectively navigate the social world. The process of developing affective competence involves coming to understand the information carried by feelings and to identify and manage emotional reactions so that they continue to provide useful feedback. However, psychiatric patients are more likely than most to experience being betrayed by feelings. Indeed, when "pain" or "bad feelings" come to be defined as part of a "disease" process, it can impair patients' ability to trust and to use their emotions as part of the necessary data for evaluating situations and making well-informed decisions.

In optimal circumstances, medications can function as a kind of crutch, bearing some of the weight of symptoms while the patient heals. An atypical neuroleptic, for example, may help a patient manage affective storms as she works in psychotherapy to organize and better understand the nature or meaning of her affective distress. Unfortunately, patients who deeply distrust their feelings may rely so heavily on medications that those medications can interfere with, or even substitute for, the patient's development. This is akin to the way an orthopedic patient could be hobbled if he always leaned on a crutch instead of trying to incrementally bear weight and develop strength in his leg. By turning too readily to medications when in states of distress, some patients fail to develop mature skills for coping with dysphoric affect and instead create a state of developmental arrest in which the only way to deal with distress is with medication.

> Mr. K, an 18-year-old male patient, seeks residential treatment after an altercation with his father in which both sustained physical injuries. Mr. K has a long history of psychiatric treatment that began at the age of 3 years when he was diagnosed with ADHD. Both stimulants and antidepressants tended to help him initially, but he seemed subsequently to become more agitated. By age 7 years, after a consultation with a national expert on childhood bipolar disorder, his diagnosis was revised to bipolar disorder, which he still carries at his current admission. His medication regimen includes two sedating antipsychotics, two mood stabilizers, and an α_2-adrenergic agonist. However, despite very high dosages of multiple medications, he is still prone to mood lability and anger that has left him seeking even more medication. Mr. K's goal at intake was "I want to be able to control myself better."
>
> Mr. K has long-standing social and emotional troubles. He appears emotionally immature and struggles to develop peer relationships. Likely adding to these difficulties, Mr. K has learning disabilities in a number of domains that necessitate academic accommodations and further separate him from his peers. He has been bullied and has bullied others. Verbal altercations commonly erupt into physical aggression both at school and at home. Mr. K and his family ascribe his difficulties primarily to bipolar disorder. Although he does not like his polypharmacy regimen, he believes strongly that he needs these medications to prevent himself from becoming dangerously manic and out of control. When his new prescriber suggests that he might be overmedicated and raises questions about his bipolar diagnosis, Mr. K becomes alarmed because he has taken it as a foregone conclusion that any capacity for containment belongs to the medication and not to him.

The family's reframing of conflict as a "problem of illness" rather than a "problem of living" has truncated Mr. K's development in several related ways. Perhaps most profound is the impact on his sense of agency and personal responsibility. In a normal maturational process, children come gradually to feel responsible for their actions and thus begin to develop ways of managing behavior and controlling impulses. When problematic behaviors are singularly understood through a biomedical lens, however, this experience of agency is often disrupted; it is now the doctor who is thought to be responsible (B. Belnap, personal communication, 2008). Consequently, Mr. K is generally not encouraged by others to develop self-control. Rather, when he gets upset, his immediate response is to take a dose of a sedating medication and sleep it off. In this way, medications actually substitute for development, and he is truly left with impaired skills for self-management.

In such situations, emotions may lose their functions as signals (Freud 1926/1959) and cease to provide guidance to patients. Those who have successfully navigated Erikson's developmental stage of initiative versus guilt (Erikson 1950), for example, take the feeling of guilt to mean that they should make efforts to curtail the guilt-promoting behavior. Some patients, however, take the experience of guilt or dysphoria to mean that they should go to their psychopharmacologist and reassess their medications. For these patients, such as Mr. K, it is almost as though they have ceased to have feelings that can usefully be explored, understood, and recruited in the service of development. Instead, they are left only with symptoms to be reduced and ignored. For Mr. K, the failure to develop affect competence feeds his negative self-image as one who is bad, sick, and irreversibly broken. The biologization of his troubles also contributes to a sense that improvements are attributable to medical intervention and not to his own efforts at self-control. He is thus deprived of any sense of emerging competence that could encourage further efforts to develop these capacities in himself.

The loss of affect competence in relation to long-term use of medications may be an inadvertent consequence of reliance on medications to address distress. Medications may also be used with defensive intent to undermine the signal function of affects. Patients may, for example, use sedating medications to cover feelings that provide useful but undesirable emotional information. The consequence of such intentional, albeit unconscious, emotional deskilling is that patients surrender the capacity to respond in healthy ways to important developmental challenges. Such patients may be committed to chronic patienthood because they attenuate their capacity to respond to conflict and dysphoric affects in any way but a biomedical one.

Ms. L, a meek and very agreeable 32-year-old woman, has been referred by her primary care provider for treatment-refractory major depression with anxious distress. Over the course of the past year she has tried several SSRIs and serotonin-norepinephrine reuptake inhibitors without significant benefit and has had a gradual escalation in her clonazepam dosage, from 0.5 mg to 1 mg and then to 2 mg, in divided doses. She reports that the clonazepam is very helpful and that she is content with her current dosage, occasionally taking less than prescribed. Her antidepressants, however, have been unsuccessful, leading to this referral. She reports some feelings of being overwhelmed at work and having substantial conflict at home with her husband of 5 years, who "gets frustrated a lot, but he's trying." When asked to provide

more detail about this conflict, Ms. L describes an unending stream of belit-
tling comments and episodic angry outbursts duruing which she is physically
intimidated, "but he never does anything to hurt me." When her prescriber
inquires whether some individual or couples therapy might also be beneficial,
she emphasizes that her husband is "working on it" and declines the offer.

Ms. L's prescriber adds an atypical neuroleptic with antidepressant properties to her medication regimen. Although Ms. L reports that it is "somewhat helpful," there is little change in her symptomatic ratings. Only after
several sessions, when she offhandedly reports taking her atypical neuroleptic in the late afternoon, does it become apparent that she is not using her
clonazepam as agreed. Given that the bulk of her anxiety is occurring in the
early evening, she is often saving her morning dose and taking a double dose
in the late afternoon. Although she is seemingly unaware of this connection,
it becomes apparent that Ms. L is taking her medication around the time her
husband comes home from work.

In this case, Ms. L appears to be using her clonazepam to mask profound
problems in her marital relationship. In the evenings, she is sufficiently tran-
quilized and therefore does not feel particularly distressed by her husband's
verbal abuse and violent threats. However, her situation is fundamentally de-
pressing. It seems likely that her mood difficulties will not improve unless
she and her husband are able to shift their pathogenic dynamic or end the
relationship. As long as she uses clonazepam to avoid facing this reality, her
depression is likely to remain recalcitrant to treatment.

When Medications Replace People

Patients may develop very deep, powerful, and dependent relationships with
their medications. For some patients, the medications may come to be more
important to them than any single person in their lives. This is especially
likely for patients with early experiences of unreliable caregiving and pronounced defenses against dependency or those who are particularly intolerant of interpersonal frustrations. As a consequence, they often expect others
to be disappointing or unpredictable and may readily turn to medications (or
other substances) in an effort to avoid the emotional risks associated with
turning to others for care. For these patients, medications are predictable,
available, and under their control, and they are able to avoid intense dysphoria
and escape interpersonal conflict, at least in the short term. However, using
medications in this way is likely to lead to long-term developmental harm. For
instance, these patients may fail to develop adequate social support systems
or the emotional skills necessary to tolerate the ambiguity and ambivalence
inherent in human relationships. They may become trapped in a vicious circle of dependence on medications and social alienation. Increasingly isolated,
their distress mounts, which increases their reliance on medications, leading

to further depopulation of their social world. If prescribers only attend to these patients' symptomatic distress, they risk missing relevant psychosocial factors and countertherapeutic uses of medications and may ultimately become unwitting accomplices in the patients' treatment resistance.

When patients develop such deep attachments to medication that it is turned to serve defensive functions, the medication may become psychologically organized as a fetish object for the patients, and its intended effect is eclipsed. A perverse process develops whereby the goal of pharmacotherapy is no longer to have health (and ideally to transcend the need for medication) but to have the medication. Contrary to the intent of treatment, such patients may keep themselves sick to secure continued access to the fetishized medication.

Medicine and Masochism

Just as it should not be taken for granted that patients are allies of prescribers, it should also not be taken for granted that patients do not want to be harmed by medical treatments. In fact, in many possible scenarios patients may desire, consciously or unconsciously, to be harmed by treatment. When such masochistic dynamics are at play, treatment resistance is a likely outcome. As described earlier in this chapter, patients who are ambivalent about illness may not only resist medications but may also recruit medications in the service of their illness. Rather than remaining ill to receive medications, these patients receive medications to remain ill. This may be because the patient obtains some concrete benefit from being ill (or being made ill), such as eliciting caregiving or eliciting guilt in caregivers or prescribers, who may then feel easier for the patient to control. On the other hand, it may reflect patients' insistence on being punished to extirpate their own guilty feelings. Even more complexly, in accordance with the principle of multiple functions (Waelder 1936/2007), the most recalcitrant symptoms (including symptomatic use of medications) may be serving multiple functions simultaneously; in this case, a patient's masochistic use of medications could serve to secure secondary gains of illness and to punish the self for this behavior, as well as serving other functions.

> Mr. M is a 32-year-old man with a history of depression and anxiety dating back to adolescence. He smokes cannabis when he can afford it and occasionally drinks alcohol to intoxication when socializing with acquaintances on weekends, but he otherwise seldom leaves his parents' home, where he has lived in a basement apartment for the past 7 years. His relations with his stepfather and mother are quite strained, as they have been since his youth. His stepfather, whom he describes as a "true bastard in every sense of the word" is perpetually angry, demeaning, and provoking, and he thinks his mother is

a "nonpresence" who "doesn't really give a shit about anything." The more pressure they put on Mr. M, the more he hunkers down into a passive and defeated position, much to their consternation. Still, they persist in pushing because the alternative solution of ignoring him has not seemed helpful either. After much effort, he has finally agreed to see a psychiatric provider, although from past experience he does not expect to find treatment helpful.

In reaction to repeated failures in caregiving early in his life, Mr. M may expect that others will be unhelpful at best and potentially quite harmful at worst. In response, he appears to manage his frustrated longing to be effectively cared for by ragefully devaluing his caregivers. Indeed, this may represent Mr. M's best effort at preempting future disappointment and wordlessly demonstrating his caregivers' harmfulness. Further still, he may secretly rejoice in his parents' injurious behavior because it helps him place the blame squarely on them and to disavow any responsibility for the ways he has vengefully contributed to the ruination of his own life. These dynamics likely underlie the perpetual control struggle with his parents, whereby he passive-aggressively provokes his parents at every turn and collapses further in the face of their response. Given this history, Mr. M's treater should expect that these dynamics will also play out in the treatment.

> Mr. M first accepts a prescription for an SSRI, which may lessen his anxiety but also further seems to sap him of desire. Pornography loses its luster, he stops going out with friends, and his self-care worsens. However, he does not directly disclose these symptoms; rather, he hints at these difficulties while covertly enjoying the demonstration of his prescriber's cluelessness. When the prescriber adds an atypical neuroleptic, Mr. M is deenergized further and begins to gain weight. Again, he only obliquely hints at these problems and, it is later discovered, takes contemptuous pleasure in his prescriber not recognizing his hints. Ultimately, Mr. M re-creates a relationship with his prescriber similar to that he has with his parents. Unconsciously motivated to focus on his doctor's failures in order to bolster his own defensive "sour grapes" position about caregiving and even to derive a vengeful pleasure from exposing his caregiver's inadequacies, he maneuvers his prescriber into surreptitiously harming him and deepening his treatment resistance.

When the doctor's unconscious resonates with the patient, the doctor may be induced to unwittingly engage in an enactment that re-creates a dynamic from the patient's past (Plakun 2003). The requirement to act (prescribe), often under time pressure and with limited information about the patient's dynamics, provides fertile ground for such enactments. Psychopharmacologists may experience feelings of inadequacy that they attempt to counter by more aggressive prescribing. This can result in complicated and potentially harmful medication regimens, especially if a patient does not tell the prescriber about worsening side effects. In this way, the patient's negative transference expectations are actualized when, ultimately, the medications produce more harm than good. Until the prescriber appreciates that the patient may have perverse (in addition to healthy) motivations for treatment, enactments of this sort are quite difficult to identify and ameliorate.

Family Dynamics and Treatment Resistance

Many of the individual-level dynamics described in this chapter may also play out within the family system. From this perspective, patients' difficulties may represent secondhand resistances that have been passed down from previous generations. To diagnose such problems, doctors should inquire about family attitudes regarding and experiences with psychiatric treatment (Table 6–2) if these have not already been offered in the exploration of the patient's attitudes about treatment.

A family's history with medications and psychiatric treatment may create powerful ambivalence and resistances that are passed on to the patient. For example, families commonly experience a member's need for treatment as a narcissistic affront and react to medications as unbearably stigmatizing (Sher et al. 2005). The patient, then, is caught in a loyalty bind between the prescriber and the family and ultimately is forced to metabolize the family's stigmatization if he or she chooses to continue treatment. When diagnoses or specific medications lead to an identification between the patient and relatives who hold negative projections within the family system (e.g., a "crazy uncle" who was also diagnosed as bipolar) or with histories of adverse outcomes (e.g., a family trauma of completed suicide while taking medications), patients may resist treatment to refuse such pathogenic associations.

Alternately, families may also hamper a patient's recovery if they unconsciously need that person to serve the role of "identified patient" for the family. For instance, in situations in which imperfection cannot be tolerated, a family system may unconsciously work to localize all troubles in one family member to relieve the other members of distress. Single mothers with troubled children, for example, are often faced, in our culture, with a dilemma: are they seen as "bad mothers," or do they have "sick children"? Evidence suggests that the usual choice is to have a sick child (Singh 2004). Although the problem is likely quite complicated and shaped by larger pathological social dynamics, the prescription serves concretely to localize the pathology in the one who is taking the pill (i.e., the child), relieving the mother (and society) of the burden of badness.

Such patients may develop treatment resistance when they acquiesce to, or rebel against, the burden of a whole-family pathology. Such was the case with Mr. B, described in Chapter 5, whose mother inquired if he had taken

Table 6–2.   Example questions to assess family contributions to
              treatment resistance

How does the family react to the diagnosis and need for treatment?
Does the family stigmatize mental health issues or medications?
Are there negative experiences with medications or mental illness in the family
  history?
What does the patient's mental illness mean to the family?

his medications every time he objected to her behavior. Mr. B faced a difficult dilemma when his medications were used by the family in countertherapeutic ways. He could acquiesce in an effort to spare his mother's fragile
narcissism and avoid escalation of conflicts, or he could refuse the role of
identified patient, leading him to fight helpful treatments. Treatment resistance may also develop in such cases when biomedical interventions fail to
address the spectrum of psychosocial stresses that may be the underlying
source of the difficulty. Furthermore, in placing all of the healing capacity in
the one who provides the pills, the patient cannot benefit from shared learning with family who have disavowed relevant personal experience.

Family systems may also medicalize problems as a defense against conflict within the family. To name a problem as medical may serve to shift responsibility from family members onto the doctor, thus freeing the family of
having to sort out complicated issues of moral judgment, choice, and personal limitation. When families fall into such a defensive arrangement, however, it may have several adverse consequences for the index patient.

> Mr. N is a 17-year-old high school junior referred for evaluation of a 6-month-
> long depressive episode that has not responded to several first-line antide-
> pressant treatments in different classes. Although this is the first time he has
> received treatment for depression, Mr. N believes he has been somewhat de-
> pressed since fifth or sixth grade and has felt anxious for as long as he can
> remember. Until this episode, he has been a highly accomplished student, in
> the tradition of his high-achieving family. Taking psychostimulants since the
> fourth grade, he overcame ADHD to achieve an A average in mostly honors
> classes while also participating in varsity sports, several social service orga-
> nizations at school, and a number of academic clubs. However, within the
> past 6 months, his grades have plummeted, and he has withdrawn from all
> extracurricular activities. Midway through the year, he was notified that he
> may not advance to the next year because of multiple school absences.
>
> When asked what he might lose if treatment were to succeed, it became
> clear that Mr. N's depression has covertly given him a reprieve from years of
> anxiously pushing himself to the edge of his capacities in order to meet his
> family's expectations. Although he is filled with despair in relation to his cur-
> rent collapse, it is not quite equal to the despair he feels at what he imagines

will be a life of anxious and unremitting toil. As long as he, his family, and the doctor agree that the problem is primarily biological, he can both rest and be spared his family's judgment for his diminished effort. Similarly, his family is spared from looking at their contributions to his feelings of overwhelm.

Although the diagnosis of major depression is uncontroversial, the family's singularly biomedical focus obscures the complicated and conflictual dynamics that have potentially led to treatment resistance. What is lost is an opportunity to empower both Mr. N and his parents to reevaluate their expectations in a way that might allow him to more easily to give up the sick role and take up the task of development in a way that acknowledges who he is and what his ordinary limitations are.

In cases in which psychological resistances to recovery contribute meaningfully to treatment resistance, a psychodynamic formulation that seeks to understand how that resistance represents a solution for the patient is beneficial to the prescriber in many ways. A deeper understanding of treatment resistance can help preserve empathy for patients and help prescribers not be drawn into collusion with countertherapeutic trends in their patients. Most important, it begins to suggest strategies for addressing the treatment resistance.

Key Points

- Treatment resistance *from* medications occurs when medications are turned, often unconsciously, to serve countertherapeutic ends.

- Patients who are treatment resistant *from* medications may be quite attached to their medications and often report symptomatic benefit but typically do not demonstrate corresponding improvement in functioning.

- Medications can interfere with functioning when they serve defensive functions (either for patients or the people around them), substitute for healthy capacities, or replace relationships.

- When medications serve major defensive functions, psychiatric chronification may result.

- Developmental arrest related to defensive uses of pharmacotherapy may often be addressed at the level of meaning and does not necessitate treatment discontinuation.

References

Erikson E: Childhood and Society. New York, Norton, 1950

Erikson E: Identity and the Life Cycle. New York, International Universities Press, 1959

Erikson E: Identity: Youth and Crisis. New York, WW Norton, 1968

Freud S: Inhibitions, symptoms and anxiety (1926), in Standard Edition of the Complete Psychological Works of Sigmund Freud, Vol 20. Translated and edited by Strachey J. London, Hogarth, 1959, pp 75–175

Glover E: The therapeutic effect of inexact interpretation: a contribution to the theory of suggestion. Int J Psychoanal 12:397–411, 1931

Husa AP, Moilanen J, Murray GK, et al: Lifetime antipsychotic medication and cognitive performance in schizophrenia at age 43 years in a general population birth cohort. Psychiatry Res 247:130–138, 2017 27888683

Kemp JJ, Lickel JJ, Deacon BJ: Effects of a chemical imbalance causal explanation on individuals' perceptions of their depressive symptoms. Behav Res Ther 56:47–52, 2014 24657311

Mintz D: Recovery from childhood psychiatric treatment: addressing the meaning of medications. Psychodyn Psychiatry 47(3):235–256, 2019 31448987

Nevins DB: Psychoanalytic perspectives on the use of medication for mental illness. Bull Menninger Clin 54(3):323–339, 1990 2207466

Plakun EM: Treatment-refractory mood disorders: a psychodynamic perspective. J Psychiatr Pract 9(3):209–218, 2003 15985933

Sher I, McGinn L, Sirey JA, et al: Effects of caregivers' perceived stigma and causal beliefs on patients' adherence to antidepressant treatment. Psychiatr Serv 56(5):564–569, 2005 15872165

Singh I: Doing their jobs: mothering with Ritalin in a culture of mother-blame. Soc Sci Med 59(6):1193–1205, 2004 15210091

Solbakken OA, Hansen RS, Monsen JT: Affect integration and reflective function: clarification of central conceptual issues. Psychother Res 21(4):482–496, 2011 21623546

Sullivan MD, Katon WJ, Russo JE, et al: Patient beliefs predict response to paroxetine among primary care patients with dysthymia and minor depression. J Am Board Fam Pract 16(1):22–31, 2003 12583647

Waelder R: The principle of multiple function: observations on over-determination. 1936. Psychoanal Q 76(1):75–92, discussion 93–117, 119–148, 2007 17294824

Wong PS: Anxiety, signal anxiety, and unconscious anticipation: neuroscientific evidence for an unconscious signal function in humans. J Am Psychoanal Assoc 47(3):817–841, 1999 10586402

CHAPTER 7

The Prescriber's Contribution to Treatment Resistance

I will follow that system of regimen which, according to my ability and judgment, I consider for the benefit of my patients, and abstain from whatever is deleterious and mischievous.

—Hippocrates

Although the term *treatment resistance* helps retain the older psychodynamic concept of resistance and implies that treatment failure may be the result of some conscious or unconscious activity on the part of patients, it is essential to recognize that doctors may also contribute in unintentional or unconscious ways to patients' poor response to psychiatric treatment. Just as patients bring their own blind spots, ambivalences, and valences for attachment and aggression, among other factors, the same is absolutely true of prescribers. A thorough assessment of the dynamics of treatment resistance also depends on prescribers being able to consider their role in the problem and to listen to the ways that their patients offer both direct and veiled feedback about the prescribers' participation in the problem.

Unconscious Collusion With Treatment Resistance

In the case of treatment resistance from medication, the prescriber, by providing medications or understandings that are turned to serve countertherapeutic ends, is recruited to serve the dynamics of treatment resistance as an unwitting collaborator. Particularly when they primarily think of medications as simple biological agents, prescribers may be unaware of the complicated dynamics underlying pharmacological treatment resistance. In addition to understanding and assessing how medications target symptoms, they must also attend to how the medications may deleteriously affect patients' overall functioning. Such was the case for Mr. K (Chapter 6), whose prescriber was swept up into the family defense, overprescribing to serve the family's powerful need to project all family troubles onto the identified patient.

Adverse Effects of Biomedical Explanations

Operating from a biomedically reductionistic perspective can exacerbate or even spark treatment resistance in other ways as well. In recent years, biomedical explanations of psychiatric difficulties have become the dominant paradigm in Western psychiatry, regardless of an ideological commitment to a biopsychosocial model. Such medicalization (Conrad 2007) has occurred not only because of optimism about advances in neurobiological science or the profound influence of drug marketing (Conrad and Leiter 2004; Moynihan et al. 2002) but also out of an earnest effort to reduce the stigma of mental illness that interferes with patients accessing crucial mental health care (U.S. Department of Health and Human Services 1999). How prescribers talk to patients about the nature of their troubles may have far-reaching consequences. When psychiatrists promote a model of patients' troubles as being primarily biological or a "chemical imbalance," they may do so for good reasons: to counter the self-blaming masochism of the patient with depression, to invoke medical authority in order to make a patient more amenable to accepting medications, or to position a patient to have an optimal placebo response. Unfortunately, patients are equally likely to be disempowered by such explanations, which invest a disproportionate amount of the power to heal in the prescriber and the prescriber's medications.

One way that patients are harmed by reductionistically biomedical explanations is, paradoxically, by worsening stigma. Indeed, stigma is multifaceted, and biomedical explanations, although offering some benefits, do not have a predominantly desirable effect on stigma (Pescosolido et al. 2010). Although such explanations do seem to reduce blame for some patients with mental illness, treating mental illness "as a disease like any other" increases the perception that people with mental illness are dangerous and unable to control themselves because they are controlled by their biology (reviewed in Kvaale et al. 2013). Biomedical explanations of illness also have the effect of increasing social difference, so that nondiagnosed people are less willing to associate with someone with a biologically based mental illness. In essence, biomedical explanations create a sense of biological otherness.

Stigma, in turn, has adverse consequences that can contribute to worsening outcomes (Sirey et al. 2001a, 2001b). People who experience psychiatric treatment as stigmatizing are much less likely to take their prescribed medications, often resulting in treatment resistance through nonadherence (Sirey et al. 2001a, 2001b). Such stigma also complicates the social lives of patients, leading to social distance that can affect important aspects of a functional life, including employment and romantic partnerships. This not only becomes a direct cause of worsening functioning but also feeds back into feelings of hopelessness and disbelonging, which only exacerbates depression and often has negative effects on health behaviors.

Patients with depression (at least mild to moderate depression) have better antidepressant outcomes when they view their depression as psychosocial in origin rather than biological (Sullivan et al. 2003). Not only is there a stigmatizing societal effect of biomedical explanations, but there also appears to be a self-stigmatizing effect. As described in Chapter 2, evidence suggests that patients who are given a biological explanation of depression are negatively affected in ways known to promote adverse outcomes. In a study by Kemp et al. (2014), participants who were told that their depression was caused by a "chemical imbalance" reported more pessimism about their overall prognosis compared with control subjects and were less likely to perceive nonpharmacological treatments (e.g., psychotherapy) as credible and effective. Not only did the knowledge that one's depression was chemically based fail to reduce feelings of stigma or self-blame, but, relative to control participants, these participants reported feeling less confident that they could effectively manage their moods (Kemp et al. 2014).

Treatment resistance may also emerge in patients in direct response to biomedically reductionistic treatments. As Fowler et al. (2011) noted, resisting treatment may be patients' best effort to confront the dehumanization and disempowerment implied in a reductionistically biomedical approach to psychiatry. In the patients' unconscious logic, to refuse medications (or refuse to be helped by medications) is to refuse to be reduced to the level of neurotransmitters, to refuse to have one's symptoms stripped of meaning and reinterpreted as the mere fallout of disordered neurochemistry. This is not to say that a psychologically reductionistic perspective does not also pose similar risks to patients. As Arnold Cooper (1985) pointed out in his seminal paper "Will Neurobiology Influence Psychoanalysis?", a one-sided focus on patients' unconscious agency in generating symptoms can be harmful as well. For example, focusing only on psychosocial factors may foster masochistic self-blame. The strength of psychodynamic psychopharmacology and other patient-centered biopsychosocial approaches is that they recognize how patients' symptoms can be determined by neurochemistry while *also* recognizing that patients have internal resources that can be recruited to either serve the functions of the symptoms or to counter them.

Confirming Negative Transferences

Prescribers may also promote transference resistance in the way they engage patients. Transference resistances occur when patients' resistance manifests as a countertherapeutic response to the doctor rather than the treatment. The result is that the treatment is undermined. Although patients can and do bring their own negative transferences into treatment in ways that thwart desirable outcomes, prescribers can certainly make their own contributions toward exacerbating a negative transference. What kind of behaviors will spark a negative transference depends, to some extent, on the particular patient. For example, neglecting the human dimension of psychiatric illness may confirm preexisting negative expectations of caregiving. Feeling treated as something less than human can easily turn patients against a prescriber. The current treatment environment—in which patients are tightly scheduled into "15-minute med checks" and the encounter between patient and harried caregiver is mediated by computers—is fertile ground for such transference resistances. Thoughtfulness about the patient and treatment and actively addressing noxious aspects of the treatment environment can help prescribers avoid becoming their patients' "feared negative other" (Winer and Andriukaitis 1989). The technical approaches recommended in psychodynamic psychopharmacology (see Part III) are intended as an antidote to some of the current pressures on the pharmacotherapeutic alliance.

Similarly, failures of tact and empathy may lead patients to resist their doctors even when they do not find their treatment to be problematic. The caregiving situation evokes deep and primitive yearnings. Consequently, a patient in treatment who has been doing well may be wounded by failures of tact or empathy that the prescriber experiences as minor or does not notice at all. When so injured, these patients may strive to reestablish equilibrium through vengeful engagement in what Cooperman (1989) coined a "defeating process." In a defeating process, the patient attempts to avenge injury by defeating the doctor and aims to defeat the doctor by defeating the treatment, often going to impressive and self-sacrificing lengths in order to achieve this objective.

Enactment

Patients are not the only people in the pharmacotherapeutic relationship who have an unconscious. Owing to their own unconscious vulnerabilities, even skilled, sensitive, and dynamically savvy prescribers may get pulled into a countertherapeutic dynamic when a charged aspect of their patients' psychology interacts with a charged aspect of their own psychology (Kayatekin and Plakun 2009; Renik 1993). This can occur when the prescriber mirrors some aspect of the patient's psychology (e.g., both have an intense but unconscious need to establish control) or when an important aspect of the prescriber's psychology is the inverse of some aspect of the patient. For example, a patient with a deep-seated but unconscious need to demonstrate the inadequacy of caregiving encounters a doctor with an equally deep-seated and unconscious need to prove his helpfulness. The struggle for control or the complementary needs to help and not be helped lock patient and prescriber in an intensifying dynamic that is sufficiently charged that neither can easily step back and examine what is happening. The result is a dynamic that recreates some powerful aspect of the patient's (and the prescriber's) life.

> Mr. O is a 24-year-old man who presents for treatment after his most recent withdrawal from college. He has a long-standing history of depression and mood instability that impairs his capacity to function independently as a young adult. Although he often begins each semester filled with energy and good intentions, he quickly becomes debilitatingly overwhelmed. With little insight into his difficulties, Mr. O manages his distress by avoiding his course work. Instead, he focuses his attention on social activities, which momentarily allow him to forget his troubles for most of the semester. However, at the end of each semester, his failing grades jolt him back into the reality of his trouble. Mr. O withdrew from school after being placed on academic probation. He is currently living with his parents despite their long-standing contentious relationship. Shortly after returning home, Mr. O's mood symptoms increased, and he began to struggle to engage in basic self-care activities. In response, his parents insisted that he seek psychiatric treatment.
>
> Mr. O describes his family as "picture perfect" from the outside. However, things are anything but picture perfect from the inside. He experiences chronic misattunement from both parents and substantial pressure from his mother. Throughout his childhood, Mr. O's father was largely absent, spending long hours developing his successful business career and traveling often. His mother, on the other hand, was highly involved and focused on helping Mr. O optimize his achievement. However, as he grew older, it became clear that her investment in him was narcissistically derived; she co-opted his successes and reacted to his failures with intense shame and criticism. In time, Mr. O also came to suspect that she needed him to appear successful as a part of a cover for her alcoholism.
>
> Mr. O presents as confused young adult who is filled with rage and highly reactive to authority. To mask his dependent longings and preempt future disappointments, he assumes an oppositional and sometimes devaluing stance toward caregivers, especially if he feels narcissistically exploited or controlled. His psychiatrist, Dr. W, also has a mother with alcoholism who had been chronically depressed and had struggled to manage as a single parent after she and his father divorced. Like Mr. O, Dr. W has had little contact with his father, who moved out of state after the divorce. Dr. W was an extremely attuned and sensitive child and sensed the increased burden this placed on his mother. In an attempt to lessen his mother's struggle and secure more time with her, Dr. W had worked to be as helpful as possible, but his efforts were

often in vain because of the limits of what he could do as a child. As he grew older, Dr. W's need to feel helpful to others had transferred to most of his interpersonal relationships, and for much of his life, this strategy has paid off, propelling him through medical school as a responsible and principled student and physician. Only recently has he begun to understand, through his own therapy, that this strategy frequently leaves him feeling depleted and privately resentful when his sacrifices in close personal relationships go unacknowledged.

By the time Dr. W begins working with Mr. O, Mr. O has failed to respond to several treatments for depression and presents with increasing desperation and anger about the failures of his treatments. The medication regimen of a serotonin-norepinephrine reuptake inhibitor, dopaminergic antidepressant, and atypical neuroleptic, with low-dosage lithium as an augmenting agent, produces only short-lived benefits, while intolerable side effects (including a 25-lb weight gain, decreased libido, and lithium tremor) have accrued. Dr. W considers adding a psychostimulant as an antidepressant adjunct to help boost Mr. O's energy levels and regulate his appetite.

In situations such as this, when the prescriber and patient have similar unconscious conflicts, it is crucial that the prescriber gain awareness about the ways in which his or her defensive processes become mobilized in the treatment. Otherwise, unrecognized enactments may ensue and disrupt, if not completely corrupt, the work. In this example, Mr. O complains bitterly about his depression. However, his focus on how his doctors have failed him unconsciously provides Mr. O with deep gratification; this both bolsters his familiar "sour grapes" defense and provides some vengeful pleasure at exposing his caregivers' inadequacy. Unable to tolerate the unspoken recrimination by Mr. O, Dr. W prescribes an ever more complicated and increasingly irrational regimen. However, the increasingly heroic efforts by Dr. W are experienced, unconsciously, by Mr. O as a repetition of his mother's narcissistic investment in his success and ultimately amplify his defensive efforts. Dr. W notices how anxious he feels before appointments with Mr. O and brings this experience to his own therapist who, over time, helps him better understand the unconscious dynamics that underlie this enactment.

Enactments can be insidious, and in cases of pharmacological treatment resistance, prescribers should be alert to the possibility that they have become unwitting participants. When the treatment-resistant patient evokes strong feelings in the prescriber, this is a sign that the prescriber may be participating in an enactment. These feelings could be either negative (e.g., angry, rejecting, or sadistic impulses) or positive (e.g., rescue fantasies, loving feelings). Similarly, prescribers may note departures from their characteristic ways of working (e.g., heroic efforts or uncharacteristic prescribing behaviors) as signs of enactment. Recognizing these signs allows prescribers to step back and initiate efforts to repair any relational damage from participation in the enactment. Having a psychodynamic formulation of their patients may also help prescribers see how their own behavior complies with well-established transference expectations in their patients. Although prescribers may be able to identify signs of an enactment and correct their position, it is often also helpful in such circumstances for these prescribers to seek consultation themselves.

Key Points

- Biomedically reductionistic explanations of illness may serve iatrogenic functions, reducing hope and a personal sense of agency and self-efficacy.

- Failures of tact, respect, and empathy can confirm negative transferences and spark resistance.

- Unconscious enactments may interfere with the rational use of medications when aspects of the patients' unconscious needs interact with or evoke corresponding unconscious factors in prescribers.

- Practicing a psychodynamically informed approach to pharmacotherapy positions prescribers to better recognize their own contributions to negative transferences.

References

Conrad P: The Medicalization of Society: On the Transformation of Human Conditions Into Treatable Disorders. Baltimore, MD, Johns Hopkins University Press, 2007

Conrad P, Leiter V: Medicalization, markets and consumers. J Health Soc Behav 45(suppl):158–176, 2004 15779472

Cooper AM: Will neurobiology influence psychoanalysis? Am J Psychiatry 142(12):1395–1402, 1985 4073300

Cooperman MC: Defeating processes in psychotherapy, in Psychoanalysis and Psychosis. Edited by Silver AS. Madison, CT, International Universities Press, 1989, pp 339–357

Fowler JC, Plakun EM, Shapiro ER: Treatment resistance, in Treatment Resistance and Patient Authority: The Austen Riggs Reader. Edited by Plakun EM. New York, WW Norton, 2011, pp 6–23

Kayatekin MS, Plakun EM: A view from Riggs—treatment resistance and patient authority, X: from acting out to enactment in treatment resistant disorders. J Am Acad Psychoanal Dyn Psychiatry 37(2):365–381, 2009 19591566

Kemp JJ, Lickel JJ, Deacon BJ: Effects of a chemical imbalance causal explanation on individuals' perceptions of their depressive symptoms. Behav Res Ther 56:47–52, 2014 24657311

Kvaale EP, Gottdiener WH, Haslam N: Biogenetic explanations and stigma: a meta-analytic review of associations among laypeople. Soc Sci Med 96:95–103, 2013 24034956

Moynihan R, Heath I, Henry D: Selling sickness: the pharmaceutical industry and disease mongering. BMJ 324(7342):886–891, 2002 11950740

Pescosolido BA, Martin JK, Long JS, et al: "A disease like any other"? A decade of change in public reactions to schizophrenia, depression, and alcohol dependence. Am J Psychiatry 167(11):1321–1330, 2010 20843872

Renik O: Countertransference enactment and the psychoanalytic process, in Psychic Structure and Psychic Change: Essays in Honor of Robert S. Wallerstein, M.D. Edited by Horowitz MJ, Kernberg OF, Weinshel EM. Madison, CT, International Universities Press, 1993, pp 135–158

Sirey JA, Bruce ML, Alexopoulos GS, et al: Perceived stigma as a predictor of treatment discontinuation in young and older outpatients with depression. Am J Psychiatry 158(3):479–481, 2001a 11229992

Sirey JA, Bruce ML, Alexopoulos GS, et al: Stigma as a barrier to recovery: perceived stigma and patient-rated severity of illness as predictors of antidepressant drug adherence. Psychiatr Serv 52(12):1615–1620, 2001b 11726752

Sullivan MD, Katon WJ, Russo JE, et al: Patient beliefs predict response to paroxetine among primary care patients with dysthymia and minor depression. J Am Board Fam Pract 16(1):22–31, 2003 12583647

U.S. Department of Health and Human Services: Mental Health: A Report of the Surgeon General. Rockville, MD, U.S. Department of Health and Human Services, 1999

Winer JA, Andriukaitis SM: Interpersonal aspects of initiating pharmacotherapy: how to avoid becoming the patient's feared negative other. Psychiatr Ann 19(6):318–323, 1989

• PART III •

The Manual of Psychodynamic Psychopharmacology

This "Manual of Psychodynamic Psychopharmacology" is meant to provide specific treatment guidelines for recognizing and addressing treatment resistance. Importantly, this manual cannot replace sound clinical training and expertise, nor should these guidelines be followed at the expense of clinical judgment. In fact, the inherent flexibility of this approach allows for optimal integration into new and ongoing treatments and affords prescribers the ability to adapt the guiding principles to the unique dynamics of their patients. At the same time, this manual addresses a need and theme within the field to articulate and operationalize psychodynamic concepts in the service of clinical application and research. Indeed, mentalization-based therapy (e.g., Allen and Fonagy 2006), transference-focused psychotherapy (e.g., Clarkin et al. 2006), and panic-focused psychodynamic psychotherapy (e.g., Busch et al. 2012) have all found ways to ground and retain their unique psychodynamic principles within a framework that can also produce measurable behavior.

This manual breaks the task of providing patient-centered, psychodynamically informed prescribing into six major technical tasks. Each of these has specific associated attitudes, skills, and clinical behaviors, which are described in Chapters 8 through 13 and demonstrated in Chapters 15 through 19. A self-assessment checklist in Appendix 1 also lays out the specific activities performed in the practice of psychodynamic psychopharmacology.

The Six Technical Principles of Psychodynamic Psychopharmacology

Psychodynamic psychopharmacology, as a practice, is grounded in six inter-related principles that, taken together, aim to support optimal pharmaco-therapeutic outcomes by recognizing the impact of psychosocial factors on treatment outcome, treating patients as partners in the work, deepening an understanding of the dynamics that move the patients and their treatment, and lessening the impact of psychodynamic interferences with treatment. These six principles are

1. Avoid a mind-body split.
2. Know who the patient is.
3. Attend to the patient's ambivalence.
4. Cultivate the pharmacotherapeutic alliance.
5. Attend to countertherapeutic uses of medications.
6. Identify, contain, and use countertransference prescribing.

The principles of psychodynamic psychopharmacology should be re-garded as interrelated and mutually dependent. For example, it is not difficult to see how cultivating a therapeutic alliance is dependent on the other five principles. A solid alliance requires, first and foremost, an engagement be-tween two people, not between a person and a collection of disordered neu-rochemicals. Avoiding a mind-body split is central to forming an alliance in which patients are genuinely treated as partners in the work. Furthermore, to truly address their patients' wishes in treatment, prescribers must have a deeper understanding of the patients' varied and often conflicting desires. In this way, the psychodynamic approach to prescribing aims to address not only patients' most superficial desires but also the unconscious dynamics that may impede successful treatment.

For example, the patient and prescriber may easily become misaligned when the patient's ambivalence is expressed in ways that undermine the agreed-upon treatment goals or when the patient uses medications in ways that are countertherapeutic. When patients and their prescribers are uncon-sciously working at cross-purposes, it is necessary to identify hidden mani-festations of conflicting agendas so that they may move back into a working alliance. Last, prescribers' own conflicts and transferences may impinge on the pharmacotherapeutic alliance so that they are irrationally motivated to behave in ways that are counter to the agreed-upon task.

Taken together, these six principles offer prescribers guidance and structure for conducting focused medical psychotherapy aimed at facilitating optimal pharmacotherapeutic outcomes.

References

Allen JG, Fonagy P (eds): The Handbook of Mentalization-Based Treatment. Chichester, UK, John Wiley and Sons, 2006

Busch FN, Singer MB, Milrod BL, et al: Manual of Panic Focused Psychodynamic Psychotherapy: Extended Range. New York, Taylor and Francis, 2012

Clarkin JF, Yeomans FE, Kernberg OF: Psychotherapy for Borderline Personality: Focusing on Object Relations. Washington, DC, American Psychiatric Publishing, 2006

CHAPTER 8

Avoid a Mind–Body Split

If the head and body are to be well, you must begin by curing the psyche; that is the first thing. And the cure, my dear youth, has to be effected by the use of certain charms, and these charms are fair words; and by them temperance is implanted in the psyche, and where temperance is, there health is speedily imparted, not only to the head, but to the whole body. And he who taught me the cure and the charm at the same time added a special direction: "Let no one," he said, "persuade you to cure the head, until he has first given you his psyche to be cured by the charm. For this," he said, "is the great error of our day in the treatment of the human body, that physicians separate the psyche from the body." And he added with emphasis, at the same time making me swear to his words, "Let no one, however rich, or noble, or fair, persuade you to give him the cure, without the charm." Now I have sworn, and I must keep my oath, and therefore if you will allow me to apply the Thracian charm first to your psyche, as the stranger directed, I will afterwards proceed to apply the cure to your head. But if not, I do not know what I am to do with you, my dear Charmides.

—Plato, 380 B.C.E.

The work of avoiding a mind-body split in prescribers' thinking begins well before they encounter patients. Few psychiatric prescribers would espouse a purely mechanistic model in which mental illness is determined exclusively by genes and neurochemical processes and in which biological processes of illness are viewed as completely divorced from psychological and social processes. Nonetheless, prescribers often operate within treatment systems and with constraints that push them toward reductionistic approaches. Psychodynamic psychopharmacology provides a counter to such cultural, economic, systemic, and psychological pressures. It facilitates the integration of the biomedical, psychological, and social aspects of mental illness and its treatment that are intimately and unavoidably connected (Balint 1957; Engel

1977). In addition, it offers recommendations and tools for integrating basic psychotherapeutic skills into the prescribing process.

Become Familiar With All Evidence Bases

In recent decades, psychiatry, perhaps even more than other medical disciplines (Tricoci et al. 2009), has been concerned with ensuring that treatment is evidence based. In practice, this has typically meant attending to the evidence base about what treatment to administer, with little or no attention given to the question of *how* to provide treatment. As reviewed in Chapter 2, a substantial evidence base demonstrates that psychosocial aspects of pharmacotherapy exert a profound influence on treatment outcome, often exceeding the effect of the actual medication. Part of avoiding a mind-body split entails the continued work of attending to *all* evidence bases pertaining to pharmacotherapy, ensuring that prescribers are guided by the best available evidence. The prescribers' understanding of the evidence base regarding psychosocial aspects of illness and treatment may also be imparted to their patients (just as one might describe what is understood about the biological actions of medications), involving patients in an alliance that includes these understandings (see "Develop an Integrated Treatment Frame").

Consider Bio–Psycho–Social Interplay in Response to Treatment

Practitioners of psychodynamic psychopharmacology recognize that mental illness and its treatment always represent a complex interplay of biopsychosocial factors. They are familiar with the evidence bases that link meaning and medications and with a biopsychosocial perspective that knows illness expression across the range of psychiatric illnesses is influenced by psychosocial factors such as adverse childhood experiences (Anda et al. 2007). In all likelihood, the interactions between these factors are often so complex that a full understanding is likely to elude both the doctor and the patient.

> Ms. P, the 29-year-old wife of a serviceman and mother of three young children, presents to the outpatient department of a military medical center with a complaint of depression. For "some time now," she has experienced insomnia, fatigue, problems with concentration, and low mood. When asked more about her mood, she describes feeling inadequate and helpless at times but is not able to further articulate her experience. Ms. P states that her insomnia and fatigue have worsened in the past several months, and she has struggled to manage her numerous responsibilities. She expresses substantial worry that her symptoms will negatively impact her family, which represents the impetus for this treatment.

In response to her complaints, Ms. P's doctor prescribes a low therapeutic dosage of a selective serotonin reuptake inhibitor and schedules a follow-up session with her in 2 weeks. At her follow-up appointment, Ms. P reports meaningful improvement in all of her symptoms and seems satisfied with her medication. Although she initially attributes her symptom improvement exclusively to the medication, on further discussion it becomes clearer to both Ms. P and her doctor that her experience is likely more complex. Ms. P reveals that her husband reacted strongly to the fact that she needs medication for her difficulties; once she was prescribed medication, he understood that her suffering is real enough to require medical treatment, and he began offering to do the dishes after dinner and taking a more active role in getting the children ready for bed, in addition to offering other forms of support.

Why has her depression resolved? Is it because of her antidepressant, because her husband began sharing the load of managing the home, because she believes that someone (her doctor) has finally recognized her suffering, or because of any number of nonpharmacological factors? When patients benefit after the introduction of a new medication, it is impossible to know the relative contributions of the many possible factors at play. Such factors include potential impacts of the active medication, placebo effect, treatment alliance, patient expectations, and motivation for change, among other possible contributors. However, an ability to respond flexibly to both biological and meaning factors in psychopharmacology in the service of enhanced outcomes is conditioned on an ability to hold an integrated perspective that recognizes patients as both subjects (who act) and objects (who are acted upon) in treatment (Docherty et al. 1977).

Humility regarding the true complexity of patients' suffering and appreciation of their adaptive and maladaptive strivings position prescribers to have a fuller, more open and authentic engagement with their patients. Such therapeutic humility keeps patients from being reduced to simple biological objects. In place of knowing there is curiosity, and curiosity may beget more curiosity. Working in this way may lead to a less paternalistic and more person-centered engagement in which both the doctor and patient can use their expertise to better understand the patient's symptoms and treatment response. Indeed, in the case of Ms. P, it was critical to her long-term recovery for the doctor to consider both the pharmacological and nonpharmacological factors that impacted her symptoms and to understand and engage her need for a more equitable distribution of household responsibilities.

Identify Reductionistic Pressures

Avoiding a mind-body split in approaching patients may sound straightforward; in practice, it requires a great deal of vigilance and discipline. Prescrib-

Table 8-1.   Contributions to a mind-body split in psychiatric thinking

Cultural biases	Dualistic concepts embedded in Western thinking, language, and metaphors
Medical countertransferences	Patient passivity and the model of the cadaver
	The "delusion of precision"
	The "war" metaphor
	Other organizing concepts
Guild polarization	Avoiding interdisciplinary tensions
Systems pressures	Pressures from care management to think reductionistically
	Stress causing defensive oversimplification
Personal countertransference valences	*Primum non nocere,* issues of competition, control, and countless others
The patient's contribution	Presenting in a way to pull to one side of the split or the other

ers face numerous pressures to approach patients reductively (Table 8–1). These pressures find their roots in Western culture and language, a consequence of Cartesian dualism that has been deeply ingrained. Indeed, Western culture does not have prominent metaphors that regard the mind and body as one. Instead, there exists an inherent linguistic separation of "mind" and "body" and "biological treatment" and "psychological treatment." This is ironic given the fact that biological treatments are, in many ways, primarily psychological (Ankarberg and Falkenström 2008), and psychological treatments bring about major changes in the structure and function of the brain (Karlsson et al. 2010; Martin et al. 2001) and can therefore be conceptualized as biological.

The environment of care can also exert significant pressure on prescribers to think reductionistically. In work settings and treatment teams, psychiatric prescribers may be assigned a role that calls almost exclusively on their knowledge of medications. Psychiatrists may be pressured by employers to "practice at the top of their license" by focusing on prescribing while psychosocial interventions are left to other providers. Insurers, too, may focus primarily on medication changes as justification for ongoing treatment or remuneration. Other forms of pressure are not so overt. For instance, models of compensation that reward patient volume over depth and complexity of patient encounter may push prescribers to narrowly define their role as simply offering medications. Moreover, the use of symptom checklists may push prescribers to focus narrowly on symptoms in a way that obscures patients' subjectivity and complexity and their broader functional and developmental goals. Similarly, by structuring the information needed about patients and splitting prescribers' attention between patients and digital devices, the electronic medical record may serve to narrow prescribers' experience of their patients.

Prescribers also face internal pressures to think reductionistically. Under stress, people typically attempt to cope by reducing cognitive complexity (Bar-Tal et al. 2013). In psychiatric practice, in which stress is often a way of life, one way this may manifest is a self-protective effort to reduce patients to a simpler biological level. Beyond common stresses related to the work setting, individual prescribers may have idiosyncratic stress responses to particular patients.

> Dr. Q is the eldest of three children, each spaced 1 year apart in age. His mother had depression, and, living by the childhood maxim that negative attention is better than no attention at all, Dr. Q often behaved sadistically toward his two younger siblings. Left with profound shame and guilt, he entered medicine with an unconscious motive of erasing the suffering he had caused in his childhood and needing first to do no harm. Although Dr. Q is psychodynamically savvy, because of his history, he is particularly sensitive to any signs of distress in his patients, especially if he feels responsible for their pain. For example, when a patient reported adverse side effects or otherwise complained, Dr. Q reactively changed the medication, uncharacteristically stripping all meaning from what might be happening with his patient. Over time, Dr. Q has learned about this vulnerability and how it impacts his therapeutic work. As he gains insight into this personal dynamic, he is able to pause and think with patients about their experiences of distress rather than immediately reducing their symptoms to concrete biomedical causes to allay his own anxiety.

Professional pressures and guild tensions that may privilege one side of the mind-body split over the other include allegiances to a particular model of treatment (e.g., biological vs. psychotherapeutic). As a consequence, this often fosters an either/or approach that denigrates the opposing theoretical model and may create interdisciplinary conflict. When there is concern regarding "turf" between "biological" and "psychological" providers, the whole arena of the meaning of medications may fall into the gray area between disciplines. Psychotherapists may be reluctant to inquire too deeply into the meaning of medications because they regard medications as the purview of the pharmacotherapist and do not want to be seen as doing anything to impinge on that work. Conversely, pharmacotherapists may worry that to make meaning, particularly to interpret transference aspects of patients' use of medications, encroaches on the territory of the psychotherapist. When both practitioners pull back from inquiring into the meaning of medications, patients may be abandoned to the most destructive meanings and uses of those medications with no help to process pathogenic meanings attached to pharmacotherapy (Mintz 2019).

Reductionistic pressures may also come from patients. Patients who are defensively invested in the experience of not being responsible for illness behaviors (Mintz and Belnap 2006) may present their symptoms in the form of an argument for a biological explanation. For example, a patient who, when asked about his mood, says he is "anhedonic" is likely making an effort to get the prescriber to see him through the reductionistic language of DSM for reasons that may not immediately be clear.

Develop an Integrated Treatment Frame

The internal work of avoiding a mind-body split in prescribers' thinking must then be translated into an integrated way of working. The beginning of this translation is in establishing a treatment frame and agreement that emphasizes the complex interactions of mind and body in mental health care and a focus on mental health as something that is more than just an absence of symptoms.

It is important to establish the place of pharmacotherapy in patients' overall treatment, which includes recognizing that there are realistic limits to what medications alone are likely to accomplish. The aim of such a recognition is to both engage patients honestly and to reduce their passive dependency on medications, allowing them to take a more active role in treatment. This task requires thoughtfulness and subtlety, however, because prescribers do not want to undermine their patients' hope in pharmacotherapy. Rather, prescribers seek to emphasize that optimism lies not only in mobilizing the power of medications but also in optimizing nonpharmacological aspects of pharmacotherapy. Although treatment-naïve patients may prefer more optimistic messaging about the power of pharmacotherapy, more seasoned patients generally prefer when prescribers recognize that medications are not panaceas (Priebe et al. 2017). Having already experienced disillusionment, these patients prefer an honest engagement that recognizes their experience and offers new paths to recovery.

As prescribers engage patients, they provide psychoeducation about the relevant evidence bases that demonstrate how psychosocial factors affect psychopharmacotherapy outcomes. This orients patients to a new approach that emphasizes their role in the pharmacotherapeutic alliance. The nature of the psychoeducation may vary based on the interests and dynamics of the patient, including discussions of the power of the placebo effect, the treatment alliance, and the patient's expectancies and desire for change. The point is first to engage patients in forming a treatment agreement that makes it clear that the therapeutic dyad will not only consider biomedical aspects of treatment but also strive to understand how the meanings of treatment are impacting the patients' response. Deemphasizing a predominantly biological theory of illness and treatment also serves to counter prognostic pessimism (Kemp et al. 2014) and other adverse consequences of a biogenic theory of illness. As with diabetes, hypertension, or other chronic medical illnesses, the treatment contract for patients with treatment-resistant psychiatric illness should emphasize that patients have a central role in managing their disease, with the goal of maximizing their authority in relation to their illness.

Furthermore, extra attention should be paid, in the initial negotiation of this treatment agreement, to aspects of the patients' relationship to treatment that seem likely to interfere with optimal outcomes. When patients see themselves as troubled simply by disordered genes or neurotransmitters, psychoeducation might focus particularly on what is understood about the complex and multifactorial nature of mental illness and on the ways that biogenic theories of illness may worsen treatment resistance. Similarly, for patients whose treatments have been marred by discontent with the prescriber, the psychodynamic psychopharmacologist will likely emphasize the role of the therapeutic alliance in promoting good outcomes, laying the responsibility on the patient to alert the prescriber to problems in the relationship. Patients who are prone to side effects might be educated, in particular, about placebo and nocebo effects, with the aim of introducing curiosity about the nature of their adverse sensitivity to medications.

Establishment of a biopsychosocially integrated treatment frame occurs not only through education but also by showing patients a way of working. First and foremost, this involves demonstrating curiosity about patients and their relationship with illness and treatment. For example, when meeting a patient for whom a biomedical understanding appears to be an organizing concept, the prescriber might try to begin translating the deeper meanings of "biological" for that particular patient. Does it mean "meaningless, disconnected from events in the patient's inner and outer life" or does it mean "not anyone's fault," or "out of my control"? By showing interest in this way, prescribers model a way of working that does not settle for reductionistic explanations. Furthermore, having asked about patients' early life experiences, relational patterns, and reactions to and feelings about pharmacotherapy, prescribers are also in a position to begin to offer hypotheses about ways that their patients may unwittingly undermine a fuller recovery.

Throughout the work, the pharmacotherapist and patient will refer back to the basic agreement to look at the patient's struggles and response to treatment not simply as an unfolding of neurobiological processes but also as a process that makes and is shaped by meaning.

Key Points

- Prescribers often face significant pressure to think reductionistically about their patients.

- Overvaluation of the benefits of medications may inadvertently disempower patients.

- Treatments can be tailored more effectively when one recognizes that illness and response to treatment typically represent a complex interplay of biological, psychological, and social factors.

- Evidence-based practice means being familiar with and practicing evidence-based prescribing behaviors.

- A mind-body split can be manifested and perpetuated in the frame of treatment.

References

Anda RF, Brown DW, Felitti VJ, et al: Adverse childhood experiences and prescribed psychotropic medications in adults. Am J Prev Med 32(5):389–394, 2007 17478264

Ankarberg P, Falkenström F: Treatment of depression with antidepressants is primarily a psychological treatment. Psychotherapy (Chic) 45(3):329–339, 2008 22122494

Balint M: The Doctor and His Patient and the Illness. London, Pitman, 1957

Bar-Tal Y, Shrira A, Keinan G: The effect of stress on cognitive structuring: a cognitive motivational model. Pers Soc Psychol Rev 17(1):87–99, 2013 23070219

Docherty JP, Marder SR, Van Kammen DP, et al: Psychotherapy and pharmacotherapy: conceptual lenses. Am J Psychiatry 134(5):529–533, 1977 848580

Engel GL: The need for a new medical model: a challenge for biomedicine. Science 196(4286):129–136, 1977 847460

Karlsson H, Hirvonen J, Kajander J, et al: Research letter: psychotherapy increases brain serotonin 5-HT1A receptors in patients with major depressive disorder. Psychol Med 40(3):523–528, 2010 19903365

Kemp JJ, Lickel JJ, Deacon BJ: Effects of a chemical imbalance causal explanation on individuals' perceptions of their depressive symptoms. Behav Res Ther 56:47–52, 2014 24657311

Martin SD, Martin E, Rai SS, et al: Brain blood flow changes in depressed patients treated with interpersonal psychotherapy or venlafaxine hydrochloride: preliminary findings. Arch Gen Psychiatry 58(7):641–648, 2001 11448369

Mintz D: Recovery from childhood psychiatric treatment: addressing the meaning of medications. Psychodyn Psychiatry 47(3):235–256, 2019 31448987

Mintz D, Belnap B: A view from Riggs—treatment resistance and patient authority, III: what is psychodynamic psychopharmacology? An approach to pharmacologic

treatment resistance. J Am Acad Psychoanal Dyn Psychiatry 34(4):581–601, 2006
    17274730
Priebe S, Ramjaun G, Strappelli N, et al: Do patients prefer optimistic or cautious psy-
    chiatrists? An experimental study with new and long-term patients. BMC Psychi-
    atry 17(1):26, 2017 28095888
Tricoci P, Allen JM, Kramer JM, et al: Scientific evidence underlying the ACC/AHA
    clinical practice guidelines. JAMA 301(8):831–841, 2009 19244190

• CHAPTER 9 •

Know Who the Patient Is

There is no health as such, and all attempts to define a thing that way have been wretched failures. Even the determination of what is healthy for your body depends on your goal, your horizon, your energies, your impulses, your errors, and above all on the ideals and phantasms of your soul. Thus there are innumerable healths of the body.

—Friedrich Nietzsche, *The Gay Science*

When it comes to treatment-resistant patients, a good starting point is the sage advice of the 12th-century philosopher and physician Maimonides, in his *Treatise on Asthma:* "Any sick individual presents new problems. One can never say one disease is just like the other. A therapeutic axiom follows: 'the physician should not treat the disease but the patient who is suffering from it'" (Maimonides 1963, p. 89). In the case of patients with chronic or treatment-refractory disorders, illness behaviors and health behaviors often have a great impact on illness trajectory. This is well understood in primary care medicine.

Psychodynamic psychopharmacology offers a viable and effective patient-centered (Balint 1969) approach to the treatment of patients with refractory psychiatric illness. In a traditional illness- or symptom-focused approach, the prescriber asks, "*What* is this patient?" in the service of seeking diagnostic clarity and matching treatment to symptoms in a way that is grounded in empirical evidence. Knowing the clinical characteristics of the depression (i.e., its duration, severity, recurrence, clinical features, somatic sensitivities) can certainly help prescribers know *what* to prescribe for the average patient. However, this knowledge may not adequately guide doctors in *how* to prescribe for every patient, given each individual's particular history, character, and concerns. In fact, in the case of treatment resistance, this approach has generally already proven inadequate. In the practice of psychodynamic psychopharmacology, an understanding of "what" the patient is will be complemented by the crucial question "who is this patient?" (Table

Table 9–1.   Prescriber behaviors that facilitate knowing the patient as a person

Consider the patient's broader developmental aims
Obtain a developmental history
Explore the relationship to treatment
Develop an "overall diagnosis"

9–1). The answers to this question begin to offer prescribers guidance not so much about what to prescribe but how to prescribe it.

Consider Broader Developmental Aims

Questions about the patient as a person and that person's motivations reorient treatment in the direction of developmental aims in ways that go far beyond mere symptom reduction. This is particularly important because, as previously noted, patients' desires for symptom reduction may come into conflict with other developmental aims (e.g., wishes to be cared for), potentially undercutting treatment efforts. As such, prescribers and patients must work together to elucidate these complex and often unconscious factors, especially in cases of treatment resistance.

Obtain a Developmental History

A cornerstone of the patient-centered approach in psychodynamic psychopharmacology is the developmental history. Taking a complete history can provide a foundation for a psychodynamic approach to the patient's medication use. This history is not simply a detailed history of symptoms and medication trials but also a developmental history that identifies important life experiences, basic relationship patterns, areas of intrapsychic conflict, and likely transference configurations (Table 9–2). The developmental history alerts the prescriber to those characteristics in the patient that may adversely affect medication outcomes (Table 9–3). Furthermore, this understanding of the patient suggests possible adaptations to enhance outcomes. For patients with a dismissive attachment style, for example, research suggests that particular attention to good communication may obviate any negative effects on pharmacotherapy (Ciechanowski et al. 2001). These patients may also respond better to a team-based collaborative care approach (Ciechanowski et al. 2006) that can provide extended support.

A developmental history that identifies patients' important life experiences and basic relational paradigms attunes prescribers to more personally unique sources of resistance to treatment. Deep-seated conflicts about de-

Table 9–2. Elements of a pharmacotherapy-oriented developmental history

Basic relational patterns
Experiences with psychiatric caregiving
Formative life experiences, especially with caregivers
Likely transference configurations
Psychosocial consequences of biomedical or genetic characteristics
Strengths and vulnerabilities

Table 9–3. Personality and temperament factors affecting medication outcomes

Acquiescence	Fast and Fisher 1971; McNair et al. 1968, 1970
Attachment style	Ciechanowski et al. 2001, 2006; Comninos and Grenyer 2007
Autonomy	Peselow et al. 1992
Defensive style	Kronström et al. 2009
Locus of control	Reynaert et al. 1995
Neuroticism	Bagby et al. 2002; Joyce and Paykel 1989; Scott et al. 1995; Steunenberg et al. 2010
Sociotropy	Peselow et al. 1992

pendency, control, abandonment or rejection, guilt or shame, self-esteem, and so on all have the potential to interfere with the healthy use of medications. Knowing that a patient experienced her mother as highly controlling would put the prescriber in a better position to identify subtle signs that the patient was reacting to the prescriber in kind, possibly allowing the issue to be engaged before a power struggle ensues. When patients' early caregiving experiences have shaped repeating relational patterns, prescribers might predict that those patterns will also be repeated with medications. For example, a patient who longs for care but is terrified of the vulnerability of dependency tends to destroy his relationships when he begins to feel dependent on another person. Such a patient may have particular difficulty tolerating medications that are helpful because it may evoke disturbing feelings of dependency. If alerted to this dynamic, the prescriber can help the patient identify and work through his counterdependent impulses to stop medications that have proven helpful and thus decrease the likelihood of relapse.

Consider Cultural Influences on Illness and Treatment Seeking

Inquiry into patients' important developmental influences also includes an understanding of the impact of culture on their illness expression and relationship to medical authority. Practitioners of psychodynamic psychopharmacology need not have any expertise in cultural psychiatry, but in keeping with an approach that recognizes the impact of meaning and developmental factors, they do need to cultivate a sensitivity to cultural issues. Although it is useful to be aware of common cultural issues in psychiatry, such as medical mistrust in Black populations (LaVeist et al. 2000) or somatic expression of depression in culturally Chinese populations (e.g., Ryder and Chentsova-Dutton 2012), this is no replacement for an attitude of cultural humility and an interest in learning about the impact of culture directly from patients. One approach is to recognize patients' expertise in their own culture and to inquire directly about their beliefs and attitudes. Although patients may be conscious of cultural factors, psychodynamic psychopharmacologists must also remain open to learning about the impact of culture because cultural factors that interfere with the healthy use of medications will be enacted and illuminated in the context of the unfolding prescriber–patient relationship.

A multiplicity of cultures may also affect patients' use of psychopharmacotherapy. Beyond ethnic cultures, many subcultures may shape patients' relationship to treatment. Medical mistrust is not restricted to populations that have experienced mistreatment at the hands of organized medicine but may be a powerful factor, for example, in groups affiliated with the antivaccination movement. Patients embedded in abstinence-based recovery communities may be exposed to stigmatizing attitudes toward psychotropic drugs. Families also have their own unique culture that may, at times, have direct bearing on a patient's treatment resistance. As Tolstoy wrote in *Anna Karenina*: "Happy families are all alike; every unhappy family is unhappy in its own way." One implication of this is that unique family cultures may adversely shape patients' ability to use pharmacotherapeutic treatment, as might occur when a family values self-reliance above all else.

Assess Character Structure

Another aspect of the developmental history that may be quite helpful is a basic assessment of patients' level of character organization. The degree of a patient's ego development and superego development may be of particular interest because these factors may shape prescribing practice with potentially abusable medications (Marcus 2007). Patients with stronger ego functions will have a greater capacity to self-soothe and to tolerate distress. For patients with weaker ego functions who may feel more overwhelmed by dysphoric affects, escaping distress may take priority over other considerations, resulting in an increased likelihood of impulsive misuse of medications. Similarly, patients who have a strong but not crushing superego are guided by basic ethical principles and can more likely be counted on to adhere with in-

Table 9–4.   Psychological and attitudinal factors influencing response
to pharmacotherapy

Ambivalence about medications	Aikens et al. 2008; Sirey et al. 2001; Warden et al. 2009
Autonomous motivation for treatment	Zuroff et al. 2007
Expectations of treatment	Aikens et al. 2005; Gaudiano and Miller 2006; Krell et al. 2004; Meyer et al. 2002; Sneed et al. 2008
Readiness to change	Beitman et al. 1994; Lewis et al. 2009
Theory of illness	Comninos and Grenyer 2007; Kemp et al. 2014; Sullivan et al. 2003
Treatment preference	Iacoviello et al. 2007; Kocsis et al. 2009; Kwan et al. 2010; Lin et al. 2005; Raue et al. 2009

tegrity to treatment agreements, minimizing the risk that medications will be misused. Patients who have less mature superegos, on the other hand, are guided more by issues of pleasure and pain and less by issues of right and wrong. This increases the probability that they will misuse potentially abusable medications in the simple pursuit of pleasure, when they are under the imminent pressure of intolerable affects, or both.

Explore the Relationship to Treatment

In addition to understanding patients' interpersonal history, it is also helpful to understand their relationship with medications and treatment (Table 9–4). Inquiry into patients' conscious beliefs about medications will often elucidate potential sources of treatment resistance (Britten 1994), such as whether they expect medications to function omnipotently or are deeply skeptical about the usefulness of medications. Armed with this understanding, prescribers are better positioned to address either magical expectations that undermine patients' agency or cynicism that undermines helpful expectations, worsening the pharmacotherapeutic prognosis (Aikens et al. 2005; Krell et al. 2004).

Even more than patients' beliefs, prescribers should assess patients' feelings about taking medications and about doctors and treatment in general. Medications and treatment often carry noxious meanings for patients that promote resistance (e.g., "I am weak," "I am defective," "I am dependent"). Patients are often aware of these meanings and can alert prescribers to attend to their treatment-interfering or nocebogenic potential. Similarly, patients may attach negative feelings to doctors. Inquiring about patients' prior experiences with psychiatric care may alert the prescriber to particular sensitivities or transference propensities (e.g., reactivity to perceived arrogance, self-preoccupation, distraction, or authoritarianism). Again, this may allow prescribers to either compensate for their patients' sensitivities (e.g., slowing down for patients who are sensitive to caregivers who make them feel rushed or perfunctory) or to explicitly attend to and address signs that such transferences are evoked.

Patients, particularly those who have been relatively disabled by mental illness, are often deeply embedded in a family context. These patients carry the burden not only of their own negative associations to psychiatric treatment but also of the fears and stigmatizing attitudes of their family. When treatment skepticism is strong within the family, patients may be exposed to consistent antimedication messaging and forced to choose between treatment and family allegiances. In such cases, the task of understanding *who* a patient is extends to understanding how familial beliefs and influences may impact that patient's relationship to medication.

Develop an "Overall Diagnosis"

Having inquired about patients' developmental history, current relational patterns, and feelings about treatment, prescribers have gathered a great deal of information that may shed light on the psychosocial aspects of treatment resistance. To optimize its usefulness, this information may be organized into a psychodynamic formulation (e.g., Perry et al. 1987) or an "overall diagnosis" (Balint 1969; Weinberg and Mintz 2018) that distills this information into the central struggles that may impact patients' capacity to make healthy use of medications (Figure 9–1). An overall diagnosis, as part of the patient assessment that guides the treatment plan, is a written explication of the prescriber's understanding of how historical, intrapsychic, and interpersonal factors are likely to influence the patient's response to psychiatric treatment.

> Ms. C, described in Chapter 5, is protecting narcissistic vulnerabilities and often does so by distancing herself from potential sources of narcissistic injury. At the same time, her longing for connection, respect, and admiration has left her vulnerable to being used and abused. Consequently, she is quite anxious about any experience of dependency, and she will likely struggle with taking medications, first because they represent a narcissistic injury, and second because, if they work, she will be confronted with the problems of need and dependency, which may make her want to stop her medications.

An overall diagnosis helps place patients' symptoms and treatment response in a broader, patient-centered context and helps prescribers keep an

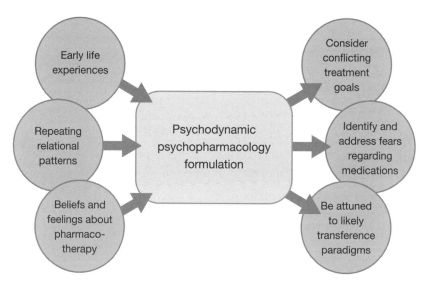

Figure 9–1.   Developing a psychodynamic psychopharmacology formulation.

eye on their patients' developmental goals while also developing a consistent framework for understanding and interpreting elements in their patients (and in themselves) that operate counter to the intended goals of treatment. As noted in Chapter 4, it is less helpful to formulate the overall diagnosis of treatment resistance in terms of pathologizing clichés, such as oral dependence, castrating mothers, immature egos, or sexual inadequacy; this is ultimately just a psychodynamic version of "illness-centered" practice. Rather, as Enid Balint (1969) noted, in the most helpful formulations the question is more one of how the patient wants to use the doctor. From the perspective of psychodynamic psychopharmacology, the overall diagnosis would include understanding of not only patients' deepest wishes for treatment but also their deepest fears.

Particularly in situations in which the psychodynamic formulation of a patient's pharmacotherapeutic treatment resistance may be rendered empathically or in which there is expectable turnover in psychiatric providers (e.g., academic centers), it can be useful to include such a provisional psychodynamic formulation in the patient's medical record. This allows the wisdom accumulated over the course of a treatment (e.g., prominent relational dynamics and defenses that complicate pharmacotherapy) to be passed on to successive providers.

Key Points

- The patient, as a person, is invited into an alliance when the prescriber considers that patient's broader developmental aims as a focus of pharmacotherapy.

- A developmental history helps prescribers anticipate and address psychosocial sources of treatment resistance.

- Alliance may be enhanced when patients believe that their prescriber is interested in them as a person.

- Understanding patients' prior and current feelings about treatment may predict and illuminate dynamics that may potentially interfere with treatment.

- A psychodynamic formulation that is focused on the dynamics related to pharmacotherapy may help prescribers anticipate patients' problems with medications.

References

Aikens JE, Kroenke K, Swindle RW, et al: Nine-month predictors and outcomes of SSRI antidepressant continuation in primary care. Gen Hosp Psychiatry 27(4):229–236, 2005 15993253

Aikens JE, Nease DE Jr, Klinkman MS: Explaining patients' beliefs about the necessity and harmfulness of antidepressants. Ann Fam Med 6(1):23–29, 2008 18195311

Bagby RM, Ryder AG, Cristi C: Psychosocial and clinical predictors of response to pharmacotherapy for depression. J Psychiatry Neurosci 27(4):250, 2002

Balint E: The possibilities of patient-centered medicine. J R Coll Gen Pract 17(82):269–276, 1969 5770926

Beitman BD, Beck NC, Deuser WE, et al: Patient stage of change predicts outcome in a panic disorder medication trial. Anxiety 1(2):64–69, 1994 9160550

Britten N: Patients' ideas about medicines: a qualitative study in a general practice population. Br J Gen Pract 44(387):465–468, 1994 7748635

Ciechanowski PS, Katon WJ, Russo JE, et al: The patient-provider relationship: attachment theory and adherence to treatment in diabetes. Am J Psychiatry 158(1):29–35, 2001 11136630

Ciechanowski PS, Russo JE, Katon WJ, et al: The association of patient relationship style and outcomes in collaborative care treatment for depression in patients with diabetes. Med Care 44(3):283–291, 2006 16501401

Comninos AG, Grenyer BFS: The influence of interpersonal factors on the speed of recovery from major depression. Psychotherapy Research 17(2):230–239, 2007

Fast GJ, Fisher S: The role of body attitudes and acquiescence in epinephrine and placebo effects. Psychosom Med 33(1):63–84, 1971 5100735

Gaudiano BA, Miller IW: Patients' expectancies, the alliance in pharmacotherapy, and treatment outcomes in bipolar disorder. J Consult Clin Psychol 74(4):671–676, 2006 16881774

Iacoviello BM, McCarthy KS, Barrett MS, et al: Treatment preferences affect the therapeutic alliance: implications for randomized controlled trials. J Consult Clin Psychol 75(1):194–198, 2007 17295580

Joyce PR, Paykel ES: Predictors of drug response in depression. Arch Gen Psychiatry 46(1):89–99, 1989 2562916

Kemp JJ, Lickel JJ, Deacon BJ: Effects of a chemical imbalance causal explanation on individuals' perceptions of their depressive symptoms. Behav Res Ther 56:47–52, 2014 24657311

Kocsis JH, Leon AC, Markowitz JC, et al: Patient preference as a moderator of outcome for chronic forms of major depressive disorder treated with nefazodone, cognitive behavioral analysis system of psychotherapy, or their combination. J Clin Psychiatry 70(3):354–361, 2009 19192474

Krell HV, Leuchter AF, Morgan M, et al: Subject expectations of treatment effectiveness and outcome of treatment with an experimental antidepressant. J Clin Psychiatry 65(9):1174–1179, 2004 15367043

Kronström K, Salminen JK, Hietala J, et al: Does defense style or psychological mindedness predict treatement response in major depression? Depress Anxiety 26(7):689–695, 2009 19496102

Kwan BM, Dimidjian S, Rizvi SL: Treatment preference, engagement, and clinical improvement in pharmacotherapy versus psychotherapy for depression. Behav Res Ther 48(8):799–804, 2010 20462569

LaVeist TA, Nickerson KJ, Bowie JV: Attitudes about racism, medical mistrust, and satisfaction with care among African American and white cardiac patients. Med Care Res Rev 57(suppl 1):146–161, 2000 11092161

Lewis CC, Simons AD, Silva SG, et al: The role of readiness to change in response to treatment of adolescent depression. J Consult Clin Psychol 77(3):422–428, 2009 19485584

Lin P, Campbell DG, Chaney EF, et al: The influence of patient preference on depression treatment in primary care. Ann Behav Med 30(2):164–173, 2005 16173913

Maimonides M: The Medical Writings of Moses Maimonides: Treatise on Asthma. Translated by Muntner S. Philadelphia, PA, JB Lippincott, 1963

Marcus ER: Transference and countertransference to medication and its implications for ego function. J Am Acad Psychoanal Dyn Psychiatry 35(2):211–218, 2007 17650974

McNair DM, Kahn RJ, Droppelman RF, et al: Compatibility, acquiescence, and drug effects, in Neuro-Psycho-Pharmacology: Proceedings of the Fifth International Congress of the Collegioum Internationale Neuro-Psycho Pharmacologicum. Edited by Brill H. New York, Excerpta Medica Foundation, 1968, pp 536–542

McNair DM, Fisher S, Kahn RJ, et al: Drug-personality interaction in intensive outpatient treatment. Arch Gen Psychiatry 22(2):128–135, 1970 4903499

Meyer B, Pilkonis PA, Krupnick JL, et al: Treatment expectancies, patient alliance, and outcome: further analyses from the National Institute of Mental Health Treatment of Depression Collaborative Research Program. J Consult Clin Psychol 70(4):1051–1055, 2002 12182269

Perry S, Cooper AM, Michels R: The psychodynamic formulation: its purpose, structure, and clinical application. Am J Psychiatry 144(5):543–550, 1987 3578562

Peselow ED, Robins CJ, Sanfilipo MP, et al: Sociotropy and autonomy: relationship to antidepressant drug treatment response and endogenous-nonendogenous dichotomy. J Abnorm Psychol 101(3):479–486, 1992 1386856

Raue PJ, Schulberg HC, Heo M, et al: Patients' depression treatment preferences and initiation, adherence, and outcome: a randomized primary care study. Psychiatr Serv 60(3):337–343, 2009 19252046

Reynaert C, Janne P, Vause M, et al: Clinical trials of antidepressants: the hidden face: where locus of control appears to play a key role in depression outcome. Psychopharmacology (Berl) 119(4):449–454, 1995 7480525

Ryder AG, Chentsova-Dutton YE: Depression in cultural context: "Chinese somatization," revisited. Psychiatr Clin North Am 35(1):15–36, 2012 22370488

Scott J, Williams JM, Brittlebank A, et al: The relationship between premorbid neuroticism, cognitive dysfunction and persistence of depression: a 1-year follow-up. J Affect Disord 33(3):167–172, 1995 7790668

Sirey JA, Bruce ML, Alexopoulos GS, et al: Stigma as a barrier to recovery: perceived stigma and patient-rated severity of illness as predictors of antidepressant drug adherence. Psychiatr Serv 52(12):1615–1620, 2001 11726752

Sneed JR, Rutherford BR, Rindskopf D, et al: Design makes a difference: a meta-analysis of antidepressant response rates in placebo-controlled versus comparator trials in late-life depression. Am J Geriatr Psychiatry 16(1):65–73, 2008 17998306

Steunenberg B, Beekman AT, Deeg DJ, et al: Personality predicts recurrence of late-life depression. J Affect Disord 123(1–3):164–172, 2010 19758704

Sullivan MD, Katon WJ, Russo JE, et al: Patient beliefs predict response to paroxetine among primary care patients with dysthymia and minor depression. J Am Board Fam Pract 16(1):22–31, 2003 12583647

Warden D, Trivedi MH, Wisniewski SR, et al: Identifying risk for attrition during treatment for depression. Psychother Psychosom 78(6):372–379, 2009 19738403

Weinberg E, Mintz D: The overall diagnosis: psychodynamic psychiatry, six-minute psychotherapy, and patient-centered care. Psychiatr Clin North Am 41(2):263–275, 2018 29739525

Zuroff DC, Koestner R, Moskowitz DS, et al: Autonomous motivation for therapy: a new common factor in brief treatments for depression. Psychother Res 17(2):137–147, 2007

• CHAPTER 10 •

Attend to Patients' Ambivalence

The patient must learn to live, to live with his split, his conflict, his ambivalence, which no therapy can take away, for if it could, it would take with it the actual spring of life.

—Otto Rank, *Will Therapy* (1936, pp. 289–290)

From a psychodynamic perspective, ambivalence and conflict are basic characteristics of mental life. Patients and doctors alike are always trying to manage their competing desires and fears. Pharmacotherapy is no different. Patients are almost always ambivalent about taking psychiatric medications (Britten 1994; Horne and Weinman 1999; Piguet et al. 2007); for example, Piguet et al. (2007) found that patients more often viewed psychiatric medications in terms of how they may harm than of how they may help.

That this ambivalence is often quite profound is no surprise given the essentially ambivalent nature of medicine. The words *pharmacotherapy* and *pharmacy* find their derivation in the Greek word *pharmakon*, which contains the dual meanings of "cure" and "poison." Even if medications do not carry a significant side effect burden, they typically represent some burden. At the very least, medications pose the burden of time, mental space, and often money. Psychiatric medications, more than many other medications, may provoke ambivalence because they also carry threats to identity and stigmatizing social meanings (Pound et al. 2005). Not being consciously ambivalent at all about medication would likely indicate some disordered relationship to medication or to health itself.

Ample evidence (Beitman et al. 1994; Kwan and Friel 2002; Lewis et al. 2009; Pound et al. 2005; Sirey et al. 2001; van Egmond and Kummeling 2002; Warden et al. 2009) suggests that significant patient ambivalence often adversely affects medication outcomes. Although it may be impossible and perhaps even unhealthy to eradicate ambivalence entirely, it is possible to

Table 10–1.   Attending to ambivalence

Assume there are areas of ambivalence

Inquire about conscious ambivalence

Listen for evidence of unconscious ambivalence

Adjust prescribing to counter negative assumptions

Interpret deep-seated pathogenic assumptions

Maintain neutrality and curiosity about ambivalence

Consider sources of ambivalence in the dynamics of the family

Explore how ambivalence impacts broader developmental aims

identify it, make it conscious, contain it, and channel it (Table 10–1). Psychodynamically informed prescribing strategies may be adjusted based on assessment of patients' ambivalence. Highly ambivalent patients whose adherence is affected by concern about side effects appear to benefit more from a start-low, go-slow approach that is "designed for comfort." Conversely, indifferent patients who neither fear medications nor expect to receive much benefit from them will need to see results to be convinced of the importance of adherence (Aikens et al. 2008). Because such patients are not especially concerned about side effects, an aggressive, "built-for-speed" approach designed to bring about a rapid response appears to be preferable (Aikens et al. 2008). Unless prescribers have assessed patients' ambivalence, this information would not be available to shape their prescribing strategy.

Explore Ambivalence About Medications

Although it would not be unusual for psychiatric prescribers to intuitively try to overcome patients' ambivalence about medications by ignoring it or by redoubling optimism, the principles of psychodynamic psychopharmacology recognize the importance of ambivalence and strive to create a safe place in which ambivalence can be brought to light, explored, respected, and engaged. The recognition that ambivalence is not only ubiquitous in both doctor and patient but also on some level derives from healthy strivings may help prescribers manage countertransference reactions when patients try, consciously or unconsciously, to fight their medications.

When inquiring about their patients' feelings regarding medications (see Chapter 9), prescribers listen not only for their fears about medically mediated side effects but also for noxious meanings the patients attach to medications that could interfere with the therapeutic effect. Although there are as many possible reactions as there are patients, it is not unusual for patients (or their family or social group) to attach stigmatizing meanings to medications such as "I am weak," "I am defective," "I am incapable," or "I am dependent." Medications may also concretely symbolize the illness experience. For example, a patient resists antipsychotics because he believes that taking an antipsychotic means that he is psychotic, and this resistance thus renders him psychotic. Patients may also ascribe negative interpersonal meanings to medications. For instance, patients may believe a prescription means there is an intolerable part of themselves that must be covered over. In such cases, medication may be equated with rejection, as was the case for Mr. H (Chapter 5), who associated the calming effects of his selective serotonin reuptake inhibitor (SSRI) with being "stifled."

Frequently, these deep-seated concerns emerge from patients' earliest or deepest conflicts. As primitive fears, they are suffused with irrationality, and the basic assumptions are so emotionally charged that they are at high risk of remaining unchallenged. When possible, prescribers work with patients to name the nature of these fears so that, in being made conscious, the fears can begin to be contained. Mr. H's pharmacotherapist eventually heard the underlying concern in the patient's repeated statements (e.g., "Oh, just put me in a cage and throw a blanket over me"). When the prescriber suggested that it sounded as though Mr. H was worried that the prescriber wanted to shut him up, Mr. H recognized this feeling and connected it with his childhood experience of being "stifled." Having already established an understanding that medication effects can emerge either from the biomedical properties of the medication or from the level of meaning, the prescriber was easily able to introduce a question as to whether the patient's expectation of being stifled resulted in the side effect of feeling emotionally blunted by his SSRI. Recognizing that this was possible, the patient agreed to restart his SSRI, and this time, the side effect of emotional blunting was gone, leaving only the desired effect of alleviating his significant anxiety, making it easier for him to engage in his psychotherapy.

Explore Ambivalence About Illness

Perhaps more insidious and difficult to treat are cases in which patient are not only ambivalent about medication but also highly conflicted about what it might mean to get better. A traditional conceptualization of medical illness takes for granted that patients' governing motivation is to get better. In cases of pharmacological treatment resistance, it is useful to consider how patients may have found covert benefits from their illness or the sick role and may be reluctant, if only unconsciously, to relinquish those benefits. Thus, it is useful to ask about their conscious ambivalence about losing their symptoms. Indeed, empathic and straightforward inquiries about what patients might stand to lose if treatment works will likely promote respect and deepen the work. If patients are aware of any secondary gains they receive from their illness, this may open a discussion of the true struggles involved in getting better and provide a grounding for the doctor and patient to struggle together with the patient's ambivalence.

> Ms. R presents for treatment of depression complicated by superficial self-harm. She is barely able to care for her 20-month-old daughter and has been unable to return to work. Her depression began after the immediate postpartum period, about 14 months earlier. Ms. R has already failed a half-dozen antidepressant trials. When asked during the course of the initial evaluation what she might stand to lose if treatment worked, she responds that she would potentially lose the caretaking attention of her husband. Judging that a competitive struggle with her infant daughter for her husband's attention is a sensitive topic that may potentially conflict with Ms. R's recovery, the prescriber informs the therapist of this dynamic, and the therapist engages the issue in their ongoing work.

Timing is often an important factor for asking such questions. The question of what the patient might lose if treatment works is best asked very early in treatment (e.g., during the first one to three sessions), when it comes from a place of curiosity and is more likely to be heard nondefensively by the patient. If the prescriber asks this question only after becoming frustrated by the patient's apparent treatment-interfering behaviors, then it will have a very different meaning between the prescriber and the patient. The patient will rightly hear the question as a challenge and respond defensively.

When patients have minimal awareness of how they have become committed to their symptoms, it often only becomes clear over time as the doctor picks up clues about the nature of the treatment resistance. Recognizing the significant role of ambivalence in treatment, psychodynamic psychopharmacologists listen for hidden benefits attached to symptoms. As noted in Chapter 5, patients may become attached to symptoms that serve important defensive functions, relieve them of onerous burdens, evoke caregiving, or serve to communicate elements of their experience that are not yet put into words. When patients derive covert benefits from illness, a referral to psychotherapy (if they are not already in psychotherapy) may provide the necessary space to explore the nature and costs of their ambivalence.

Maintain Relative Neutrality About Symptoms When Conflicts Arise

The position prescribers take in relation to patients' symptoms and ambivalence is important. Often, patients are unconsciously invested in protecting their symptoms, even at great personal cost. Thus, prescribers must be careful not to take too strong a stand about the symptom. Indeed, challenging it too forcefully may risk provoking further defensive maneuvers, entrenching the symptom further. In this case, the patient no longer believes the doctor is in alliance with his or her true wishes, increasing the patient's resistance. It is not the pharmacotherapist's place to decide health is preferable to the benefits offered by illness. In psychodynamic psychopharmacology, a neutral position that does not take sides but instead expresses curiosity and respect for the difficult dilemmas patients are facing allows them to bring the conflict into fuller view, in which the actual costs of the solution may be explored, possibly shifting patients toward readiness to change.

> Mr. S, a 19-year-old man, presents to treatment for myriad mood symptoms accompanied by intrusive, violent mental images and some minor contamination concerns. He has experienced, at best, partial responses to SSRIs and clomipramine. However, the full potential of these medications is unknown given his history of poor adherence. Before this treatment, Mr. S reports a several-month depressive withdrawal during which he played video games at night and slept for much of the day. His ambivalence about getting better has become apparent, and he is working on understanding this with his therapist and discussing these dilemmas with his pharmacotherapist. Although there are several reasons he is ambivalent, the most prominent reason is that his illness appears to serve the function of saving his parents' marriage. When he is ill, they join forces to help him and function well as a pair. However, when he is doing better, long-standing resentments resurface and plunge his parents into stereotyped and escalating recriminations that have repeatedly brought them to the brink of divorce.

Should it be up to the doctor to decide that this patient's health is worth the loss of his family? Instead, the prescriber can be empathic about the dilemmas the patient faces while continuing to offer, not too forcefully, to optimize Mr. S's prescriptions and develop strategies to help with adherence.

Attend to the Family Context

Like prescribers, families may also exacerbate ambivalence. As noted earlier, when families have stigmatizing attitudes about treatment, it can fuel patients' ambivalence. Conversely, when families invest too much in medications, it can also increase patients' resistance to treatment. Struggles for autonomy are one mechanism by which a family's investment in treatment may push patients into treatment opposition. Furthermore, when families are highly invested in patients' medications, the medications often come to serve a defensive function in the family. If, for example, medications are used by the family to localize family pathology in the person taking the medications (e.g., Mr. B, Chapter 5), then it is understandable that the patient will resist medications that are cementing his or her role as the identified patient.

Often, it is sufficient for patients to understand that their resistance to medication is actually a resistance to a family dynamic in order for them to begin questioning their need to resist medications. Prescribers can aid this process by respectfully exploring the dilemma and remaining neutral about whether patients take medications. In this way, the prescriber becomes differentiated from the family and becomes usable as a resource. When the family dynamic is particularly noxious or when there are real threats to a patient's autonomy, the prescriber may choose to meet with the patient and the family to review some of the nonpharmacological factors (e.g., family dynamics) that may impact treatment outcomes.

Key Points

- Patients are almost always ambivalent about taking medications, often for good reason.

- Ambivalence should be explored rather than ignored.

- Psychodynamically informed prescribing strategies may be adjusted based on assessment of patients' ambivalence.

- Ambivalence is best addressed from a neutral stance that is empathic with a patient's dilemma.

- Unconscious sources of ambivalence to pharmacotherapy may be more effectively addressed when brought to conscious awareness (e.g., through interpretation).

References

Aikens JE, Nease DE Jr, Klinkman MS: Explaining patients' beliefs about the necessity and harmfulness of antidepressants. Ann Fam Med 6(1):23–29, 2008 18195311

Beitman BD, Beck NC, Deuser WE, et al: Patient stage of change predicts outcome in a panic disorder medication trial. Anxiety 1(2):64–69, 1994 9160550

Britten N: Patients' ideas about medicines: a qualitative study in a general practice population. Br J Gen Pract 44(387):465–468, 1994 7748635

Horne R, Weinman J: Patients' beliefs about prescribed medicines and their role in adherence to treatment in chronic physical illness. J Psychosom Res 47(6):555–567, 1999 10661603

Kwan O, Friel J: Clinical relevance of the sick role and secondary gain in the treatment of disability syndromes. Med Hypotheses 59(2):129–134, 2002 12208197

Lewis CC, Simons AD, Silva SG, et al: The role of readiness to change in response to treatment of adolescent depression. J Consult Clin Psychol 77(3):422–428, 2009 19485584

Piguet V, Cedraschi C, Dumont P, et al: Patients' representations of antidepressants: a clue to nonadherence? Clin J Pain 23(8):669–675, 2007 17885345

Pound P, Britten N, Morgan M, et al: Resisting medicines: a synthesis of qualitative studies of medicine taking. Soc Sci Med 61(1):133–155, 2005 15847968

Rank O: Will Therapy: An Analysis of the Therapeutic Process in Terms of Relationship. New York, Knopf, 1936

Sirey JA, Bruce ML, Alexopoulos GS, et al: Stigma as a barrier to recovery: perceived stigma and patient-rated severity of illness as predictors of antidepressant drug adherence. Psychiatr Serv 52(12):1615–1620, 2001 11726752

van Egmond J, Kummeling I: A blind spot for secondary gain affecting therapy outcomes. Eur Psychiatry 17(1):46–54, 2002 11918993

Warden D, Trivedi MH, Wisniewski SR, et al: Identifying risk for attrition during treatment for depression. Psychother Psychosom 78(6):372–379, 2009 19738403

• CHAPTER 11 •

Cultivate the Pharmacotherapeutic Alliance

To write prescriptions is easy, but to come to an understanding with people is hard.

—Franz Kafka, "A Country Doctor"

In addition to ambivalence about medications and illness, patients may be ambivalent about their doctors. This may emerge from transference-based expectations of caregivers, problems in the real relationship between doctor and patient, or both. Although every medical student learns that the doctor–patient relationship is of central importance in the practice of medicine, this dyad typically receives far less attention than the more "specific" treatments the doctor offers. Given that the therapeutic alliance often appears to contribute more potently to pharmacological treatment outcomes than the actual drug being used (Krupnick et al. 1996), it is essential to cultivate a strong alliance. This means not only gaining patients' respect through competence, presence, tact, and empathy but also respecting patients' capacities as participants in the therapeutic endeavor by engaging them as partners and actively confronting the conditioned distortions regarding prescribers and caregiving figures in general that they bring into pharmacotherapy (Table 11–1).

Establishing an alliance draws heavily on the other principles of psychodynamic psychopharmacology. It requires that prescribers avoid mind-body splits, not only engaging the illness but also adopting a person-centered approach that privileges patients' subjectivity and agency. This, in turn, requires that prescribers know not only *what* the patient is, diagnostically, but also *who* the patient is, as a person. A true alliance is not struck with only one part of the patient, and having a deeper understanding of patients' conflicts and ambivalences allows prescribers to ally with them on multiple levels. Prescribers are also positioned to recognize places in which patients' differing goals are irreconcilable. The alliance may then be strengthened as prescribers work

129

Table 11–1.   Evidence-based elements of an effective alliance

Agreement about targets
Autonomy support
Good communication
Respect for treatment preferences
Shared decision making
Warmth and presence

empathically with the impossibility of identifying a perfect solution. When treatments not only are undermined by issues in the patient (or doctor) but are turned to serve countertherapeutic ends, psychodynamic psychopharmacologists will identify that a misalliance (Langs 1975/1981) has formed and will work to return, as much as possible, to an overall alliance. Prescribers will also recognize that it is not only patients but also prescribers who may, in responding to their own conflicts, introduce misalliances into the work, thereby undermining optimal outcomes.

Focus on Elements of Effective and Empowering Healing Relationships

The work of forging an alliance capitalizes on "common factors" (Frank 1971; Table 11–2) that account, in large measure, for the potency of therapeutic relationships. Although common factors are most often thought of as major contributors to psychotherapeutic outcomes, they likely also play an important role in pharmacotherapy (Davidson and Chan 2014; Greenberg 2016). In addition to establishing a therapeutic relationship, Frank (1971) suggested that effective treatments will create an expectation of help, involve the active participation of both doctor and patient, and impart a rationale or conceptual scheme that explains the trouble and prescribes a given ritual or procedure for resolving symptoms.

Attend to Nonverbal Aspects of the Alliance

The work of negotiating an alliance begins the moment the doctor and patient meet. Nonverbal aspects of the initial engagement play a significant role in shaping the unfolding alliance. Warmth (Rickels et al. 1971), including in vocal tone (Cruz et al. 2013), facilitates an engagement for most patients. As prescribers begin to elicit their patients' story, they convey a sense of empathy (Downing et al. 1973) for the patients' dilemmas and demonstrate an interest in the outcome (Lyerly et al. 1964). At times, this may include time-limited alterations in the meeting schedule, with more frequent meetings

Table 11–2.　Common factors in treatment

Active participation of both doctor and patient in an emotionally charged setting

Expectation of help

Persuasive rationale or conceptual scheme that explains the trouble

Ritual or procedure for resolving symptoms

Source.　Adapted from Frank 1971.

demonstrating, nonverbally, the prescriber's commitment to the patient's treatment while affording increased opportunities for useful engagement. When possible, prescribers also attempt to minimize the intrusion of digital devices between them and their patients (Rosen et al. 2016).

Maintain a Person-Centered Focus

Prescribers establish that their focus will be person-centered by conveying interest in the person of the patient. This is achieved by eliciting the patients' stories, including important stories from their lives, and discovering their overarching developmental goals. Prescribers communicate this further as they recognize patients' values and developmental goals (e.g., to be independent or to find love) that transcend a symptom focus but will be impacted by successful pharmacotherapy. One element that differentiates the approach of psychodynamic psychopharmacology as psychodynamically informed is the recognition that patients' motivations and desires relative to treatment may well be unconscious, complex, and conflictual. As such, a fuller picture of their motivations for treatment may only emerge over time as both prescriber and patient begin to make meaning of problems that emerge in pharmacotherapy.

Support Development of the Patient's Agency

The person-centered focus of psychodynamic psychopharmacology is buttressed by the effort to engage patients' agency. This work starts with prescribers recognizing and containing various pulls into a subject-object mode of relating (see Chapter 8) in which patients are treated as biological substrates of treatment. Instead, each patient, as a person, is recognized as having a subjectivity and internal resources that can be brought to bear in the struggle against the illness.

A psychodynamic sensibility has implications for the understanding of agency. Agency is not simple and straightforward because it is shaped and delimited by the unconscious. Patients are not simply understood as having a will that can be mobilized against illness by engaging in healthy behaviors.

Instead, their thoughts are considered to have potency because factors such as positive expectations, autonomous motivation for treatment, and readiness to change all have the potential to facilitate (or interfere with) a manifestly desirable treatment outcome. Further still, patients are understood to have agency that may be mobilized in the opposite direction from "health." In the context of treatment resistance, it is understood that patients may be surreptitiously opposing treatment efforts, obeying a deeper self-protective instinct of which they may be unaware. If such dynamics are identified, their conscious agency may be marshaled to explore and confront unconscious countertherapeutic impulses, further enhancing the path to recovery.

Patient-centered approaches frequently position patients as the experts on themselves as a counterweight to providers' expertise regarding the various reasonable treatments. However, from a psychodynamic perspective, expertise about oneself is always delimited by the presence of the unconscious. At times, others may have a vantage point from which they can discern motivations that are unknown to the individual. Expertise on the self (for both the patient and doctor) is not something one simply has (as described in Chapter 3) but something that one struggles toward, with agency and self-expertise increasing to the extent that unconscious factors are brought into conscious awareness, such as when a patient comes to see that fears of dependency have interfered with effective treatment.

There are several ways in which patients' authority can be supported in the ordinary conduct of psychodynamic psychopharmacology. As in common patient-centered approaches, prescribers adopt a communication style that facilitates autonomy, self-care, and health promotion. Authoritative but not authoritarian, they educate their patients, as much as reasonably possible, about the various treatment options and the potential for adverse reactions. Although educating patients about possible side effects runs the risk of increasing nocebo responses, it also makes it more likely patients will continue their medications if any side effects emerge (Bull et al. 2002). Prescribers also educate patients about things that they can do for themselves, such as making lifestyle changes, including exercise for patients with depression, developing regular social rhythms for those with bipolar disorder, and avoiding cannabis for those with psychosis.

Patient preferences regarding treatment are elicited when it comes time to make treatment decisions. Even involvement in simple decisions, such as the dosing schedule of a medication, can enhance adherence (Woolley et al. 2010). Within the bounds of reason and conscience, patients should be offered their preferred option, ideally with an explanation of how this is the optimal treatment for them. In all likelihood, it will be optimal not because the choice is manifestly better than other options but because it is the treatment the patient wants, and evidence suggests that preferred treatments will work better than nonpreferred treatments (Kocsis et al. 2009). This explanation is part of the developing understanding that patients' subjectivity may play a major role in treatment outcomes.

This does not mean that patients' preferences should not be not questioned. Indeed, given the goal of knowing who the patient is (see Chapter 9), it is part of the task of psychodynamic psychopharmacologists to shed light on patients' decision making. Such decisions likely involve elements of irrationality (e.g., it was seen on a commercial, it is different from the treatment the patient's parent is advocating), and exploring these elements extends patients' agency by allowing them (as opposed to their unconscious) to be more in control of decision making.

Psychodynamic psychopharmacologists also support patients' agency by taking a more active role in questioning their deauthorizing assumptions. For instance, when a patient adopts a biomedically reductionistic position (e.g., insisting that a bad feeling is simply a meaningless manifestation of depression), the prescriber may want to inquire about how the patient *knows* this. In particular, attitudes that tend to strip feelings of meaning should be questioned because such attitudes can contribute to a loss of affect competence. Curious questioning that helps differentiate problems of illness from problems of living (see Chapter 17) and identifies the signal functions of affect serve further to teach patients to make use of feelings, enhancing affect competence and personal agency.

Ms. T, age 19 years, is admitted for treatment to a residential treatment program for unremitting depression with anxious distress and complex medical issues that are not well understood. She is taking several medications, including high-dosage selective serotonin reuptake inhibitors and a benzodiazepine, which is changed to gabapentin shortly after admission. In treatment, her medical symptoms are recharacterized as symptoms of somatization. One therapeutic focus is on helping her express with words what she could previously only express with her body. This reframing of a shared family defense in which her problems are medicalized, rather than understood to be meaningful and to have communicative value, creates significant anxiety in her family. After 10 weeks of treatment, they precipitously tell her that there are no further resources for treatment.

The next day, Ms. T seeks an urgent consultation with her prescriber, insisting that she be taken off of gabapentin "because it's making me angry." Based on previous experiences with prescribers, she expects to be taken at face value and believes her gabapentin will be discontinued. In this case, however, the prescriber raises questions about the obvious association between her precipitous discharge and feelings of anger. Rather than collude with a medical defense that serves to detoxify negative feelings in the family, the prescriber suggests that she first explore in her therapy whether her anger is not, in fact, a side effect but rather a reaction to the hurried way her treatment is being ended. She is then able to differentiate herself further from an enmeshed family dynamic and confront her family about the ways that avoidance of conflict often results in such abrupt decisions.

Establish Hope

Prescribers operating from a more purely biomedical framework may emphasize the potency, specificity, and precision of medications targeted to specific symptoms or neural systems. This is often done to instill hope and to enhance placebogenic expectations. However, overemphasizing biogenic explanations and the healing power vested in prescribers and their medications risks disempowering patients and, paradoxically, giving patients less, rather than more, hope (Kemp et al. 2014). Feeling stricken by a biological disease beyond their control, they may surrender personal agency, passively awaiting cure by their doctor's medications.

Recognizing that overly optimistic presentations of the potency of medications will likely not ring true to patients who have already experienced pharmacological treatment resistance, psychodynamic psychopharmacologists try to convey a more realistic stance regarding what medications can and cannot do by themselves. What prescribers convey is the hope that, by applying the principles of psychodynamic psychopharmacology, engaging patients' agency, working on the therapeutic alliance, and mobilizing other meaning-based factors known to optimize pharmacotherapeutic outcomes, treatment resistance may be reduced or even eliminated. This approach offers other forms of hope as well. Given the actual limitations of medications in the face of serious psychiatric troubles, there is no guarantee that either psychodynamic psychopharmacology or cutting-edge use of medications will effect a clinically significant improvement in symptoms. What psychodynamic psychopharmacology does offer in these situations is a recognition that solutions are always partial at best, given the conflictual nature of mental life. Patients are given hope, within a patient-centered perspective, that they will be supported in developing greater agency in relation to their illness so that personal growth may be one consequence of facing their treatment resistance. Furthermore, prescribers' recognition of the role of the person in pharmacotherapy and the role of the relationship often means that patients struggling with treatment resistance will be less alone in the struggle.

Provide a Therapeutic Rationale

Psychodynamic psychopharmacology represents a specific way of working that is a departure from the more biomedically oriented approach that has dominated psychiatry since the 1990s. The emphasis on biopsychosocial integration, patients' subjectivity, and the perspective that patients, as much as doctors, bear responsibility for treatment may represent a significant shift in what patients expect from psychiatric treatment. Part of the work of forging an alliance is finding agreement about this way of working. Patients sometimes become interested in this approach as prescribers demonstrate a person-centered approach that strives to form not only an objective-descriptive diagnosis but also an overall diagnosis that integrates an understanding of the psychosocial dimensions of the patients' life.

Prescribers optimize common factors in healing by explaining the rationale for this way of working. Educating patients pertains not only to the evidence base regarding specific medications but also to the various ways that psychosocial factors impact pharmacological treatment outcomes. This education helps position patients to engage as partners in several ways. It calls for patients to be more active participants in treatment by emphasizing their role in treatment outcome, mediated by variables such as treatment expectancies and readiness to change. By emphasizing the immeasurable complexity of mind-body interactions, it strives to induce their curiosity about the deeper causes of both positive and negative treatment outcomes, broadening the armamentarium of both the prescriber and the patient.

By emphasizing the potential potency of the therapeutic alliance, prescribers place a burden on both their patients and themselves to maintain a strong alliance in the service of optimizing outcomes. Strains on the alliance are likely unavoidable, and patients should be informed that they are permitted to voice complaints or concerns about their prescriber's way of working because such feedback is necessary for the treatment alliance to function optimally. Prescribers must become comfortable with hearing their patients' criticism and negative feelings and be able to address those feelings nondefensively. It may be helpful to remember that in any enduring relationship, injuries, however small, will always occur.

Work With Negative Transferences

Although patients' complaints and concerns should be taken seriously, this does not mean that they should be responded to immediately. It is valuable to consider whether a patient's particular negative reaction to a medication or the prescriber may be related to the activation of ingrained expectations deriving from the patient's most formative experiences. When there is evidence that transferences or repeating interpersonal patterns have interfered with patients' relational functioning, it may be particularly useful to introduce the question of transference before transference resistances have been sparked.

For example, while assessing Ms. C (see Chapter 5) during pharmacotherapy intake, it became apparent that the anxiety evoked by her dependent yearnings had caused her repeatedly to destroy relationships in order to ameliorate her anxiety. In such cases, prescribers can highlight this dynamic and predict that if treatment works, related feelings about the doctor or medication will likely be evoked. They can then engage patients at a rational level about this dynamic, alerting them to attend to subtle concerns about dependency before they succumb to a more intense state of anxiety that might render it difficult or even impossible to think.

In the course of this work, prescribers (and patients) must carefully attend to issues of transference, in the context not only of patients' consciously negative feelings about the prescriber but also of other clinically meaningful events, including missed appointments, medication nonadherence, the emergence of side effects, requests for medication changes, requests for consultation, and even the appearance of an overly compliant patient attitude. When, for example, patients develop issues with adherence to medication or treatment, prescribers may usefully inquire about whether this symptom reflects a problem in the relationship with the doctor.

Patients may adopt a position that they "know" what is happening because they know their body. Although they may be right, such pathological certainty (Shapiro 1982) should alert prescribers to the operation of intrapsychic or interpersonal defenses. Likewise, prescribers should be mindful not to fall into the position of being "the one who knows" (Lacan 1966, p. 403) regarding the transference origins of side effects or problems in the alliance. Any sense on the part of prescribers that they know the truth better than their patients should alert them that they have also succumbed to unconscious processes. For example, a prescriber may defensively disavow his role in contributing problematically to the "real relationship" by adopting behavior that undermines the alliance, such as behaving uncaringly or imperiously claiming to know the patient better than she knows herself. Worse, to "know" that the patient's "side effects" are transference manifestations may put that patient at risk of medical harm. For doctors and patients, a measure of humility about the relative contribution of transference creates a space for reflection, experimentation, and learning while avoiding reactivity.

Emphasize Alliance, Not Compliance

In pharmacotherapy, *alliance* is often confused with *compliance* (Gutheil and Havens 1979), and patients are often seen as being "in alliance" with the doctor when they take their medications. Patients may also think they have a good alliance with their doctor when the doctor gives them the medications they want, regardless of the doctor's misgivings. Alliance is a two-way street; it is a negotiation in which neither participant submits to the will of the other, and both find a way to feel invested in the treatment plan. The model of doctors as the ultimate authorities on patients' health is frequently more harmful than helpful. Similarly, it is not useful to conceptualize doctors as servants because the customer is not always right. A model of shared inquiry and partnership is ideal and appears to promote long-term adherence (Frank et al. 1995).

Key Points

- Alliance means not only gaining patients' respect through a combination of competence, presence, tact, and empathy but also respecting their capacities as participants in the therapeutic endeavor.

- Realistic therapeutic humility about the limits of medications can be coupled with realistic hope about the benefits of an enhanced alliance and integration of psychosocial factors into treatment.

- Integrating patient preferences into the pharmacotherapeutic treatment plan often enhances alliance and improves outcomes.

- Patients' agency may be supported by questioning or challenging their deauthorizing assumptions.

- Negative transferences can be addressed to help patients identify when previous negative experiences with caregiving are interfering with their current ability to make optimal use of pharmacotherapy.

References

Bull SA, Hu XH, Hunkeler EM, et al: Discontinuation of use and switching of antidepressants: influence of patient-physician communication. JAMA 288(11):1403–1409, 2002 12234237

Cruz M, Roter DL, Cruz RF, et al: Appointment length, psychiatrists' communication behaviors, and medication management appointment adherence. Psychiatr Serv 64(9):886–892, 2013 23771555

Davidson L, Chan KK: Common factors: evidence-based practice and recovery. Psychiatr Serv 65(5):675–677, 2014 24535634

Downing RW, Rickels K, Dreesmann H: Orthogonal factors vs. interdependent variables as predictors of drug treatment response in anxious outpatients. Psychopharmacology (Berl) 32(2):93–111, 1973 4584949

Frank E, Kupfer DJ, Siegel LR: Alliance not compliance: a philosophy of outpatient care (discussion). J Clin Psychiatry 56(suppl 1):11–16, discussion 16–17, 1995 7836346

Frank JD: Eleventh Emil A. Gutheil memorial conference: therapeutic factors in psychotherapy. Am J Psychother 25(3):350–361, 1971 4936109

Greenberg RP: The rebirth of psychosocial importance in a drug-filled world. Am Psychol 71(8):781–791, 2016 27977264

Gutheil TG, Havens LL: The therapeutic alliance: contemporary meanings and confusions. International Journal of Psycho-Analysis 6(4):467–481, 1979

Kemp JJ, Lickel JJ, Deacon BJ: Effects of a chemical imbalance causal explanation on individuals' perceptions of their depressive symptoms. Behav Res Ther 56:47–52, 2014 24657311

Kocsis JH, Leon AC, Markowitz JC, et al: Patient preference as a moderator of outcome for chronic forms of major depressive disorder treated with nefazodone, cognitive behavioral analysis system of psychotherapy, or their combination. J Clin Psychiatry 70(3):354–361, 2009 19192474

Krupnick JL, Sotsky SM, Simmens S, et al: The role of the therapeutic alliance in psychotherapy and pharmacotherapy outcome: findings in the National Institute of Mental Health Treatment of Depression Collaborative Research Program. J Consult Clin Psychol 64(3):532–539, 1996 8698947

Lacan J: Ecrits. Paris, Seuil, 1966

Langs R: Therapeutic misalliances (1975), in Classics in Psychoanalytic Technique. Edited by Langs R. New York, Jason Aronson, 1981, pp 291–306

Lyerly SB, Ross S, Krugman AD, et al: Drugs and placebos: the effects of instructions upon performance and mood under amphetamine sulfate and chloral hydrate. J Abnorm Psychol 68(3):321–327, 1964 14126847

Rickels K, Lipman RS, Park LC, et al: Drug, doctor warmth, and clinic setting in the symptomatic response to minor tranquilizers. Psychopharmacology (Berl) 20(2):128–152, 1971 4933093

Rosen DC, Nakash O, Alegría M: The impact of computer use on therapeutic alliance and continuance in care during the mental health intake. Psychotherapy (Chic) 53(1):117–123, 2016 26214322

Shapiro ER: On curiosity: intrapsychic and interpersonal boundary formation in family life. Int J Fam Psychiatry 3(1):69–89, 1982

Woolley SB, Fredman L, Goethe JW, et al: Hospital patients' perceptions during treatment and early discontinuation of serotonin selective reuptake inhibitor antidepressants. J Clin Psychopharmacol 30(6):716–719, 2010 21105288

• CHAPTER 12 •

Attend to Countertherapeutic Uses of Medications

The greatest disease of men arose from the fight against their diseases, and the apparent remedies have, in the long run, created worse than that which was to be eliminated by them.

—Friedrich Nietzsche

When seen from a psychodynamic perspective, mental life is fraught with irrationality. Conscious thought represents a compromise between competing wishes, impulses, demands, and prohibitions. Prescribers must come to terms with a certain degree of irrationality in their patients' use of medication, respecting patients' competing agendas. In such cases, not much needs to be done except to cast some light on the irrationality. At times, these irrational uses may be in the service of development, as occurs when patients use medications as transitional objects while they learn that the capacity for healing or self-soothing is actually within themselves. There are times, however, when a misalliance emerges that is significant enough that it must be addressed. This is especially true when patients' medications are being used to serve some serious countertherapeutic end. The principle of respecting patients' (often unconscious) authority may, in such cases, clash with a much deeper principle: *primum non nocere*. When prescribed medications become a source of covert harm, the prescriber is implicated and must decide what to do about having been induced into colluding with harming the patient with pharmacotherapy.

As detailed in Chapter 6, patients may recruit the effects of medication to serve countertherapeutic ends, such as when they use the consciousness-dulling effects of medications to avoid developmentally appropriate feelings, as was the case in that chapter with Ms. L, who used her clonazepam to avoid facing the reality of her abusive situation. Medications may also interfere with healthy development, as when patients surrender their capacity for self-management and emotional regulation to the medication, thus allowing those skills to atrophy or not develop at all (e.g., Mr. K, Chapter 6). Just as medications can be used to replace parts of the self (e.g., self-regulating capacities), they can also be used to replace people, as occurs when patients turn to medication rather than people for soothing. Often it is not the medication itself but the meaning attached to it that becomes countertherapeutic, as occurs when biomedical explanations attached to medications are used defensively to avoid self-knowledge or personal responsibility.

Identifying Countertherapeutic Uses of Pharmacotherapy

It is not always easy to identify when medications are serving subtle countertherapeutic ends and patients are experiencing a significant degree of treatment resistance *from* medications. This is particularly true when patients experience the medication as helpful and there is evidence of attenuation of some symptoms.

Think Like a Mental Health Professional

Prescribers' ability to recognize countertherapeutic use of medications may be conditioned on their conceptualization of the therapeutic task. By placing a singular focus on symptoms and symptom reduction, many providers have inadvertently become mental *illness* professionals, pursuing the symptoms while losing sight of the larger developmental aims. In this way, a patient who *feels better* with medication but does not *get better* may be seen simply as someone with a chronic illness who has benefited substantially from medications, so impediments to fuller recovery are not addressed. In contrast, a mental *health* professional is concerned not only with the absence of illness but even more with the promotion of health. By prescribing in a way that fosters patients' agency and overall adaptive capacity, mental health professionals are more likely to be attuned to the defensive and disempowering use of medications and equipped to address countertherapeutic uses and effects.

Recognize the Signs

What is complicated about countertherapeutic uses of medications is that such misuses are often not immediately apparent to either patients or prescribers. Prescribers should remember that countertherapeutic uses of medications may be quite subtle, and they should remain attentive to signs that they are being used countertherapeutically (Table 12–1). Such patients believe medications are helpful (and they are) without recognizing how their

Table 12–1. Signs of countertherapeutic use of medications

Patient feels better with medications but does not get better

Symptoms are lessened, but overall functioning does not improve

Patient appears to be becoming a chronic patient

Patient appears attached to medication or to associated diagnoses

Patient defensively uses diagnoses to avoid personal responsibility

Patient uses medications to avoid developmentally appropriate feelings

Prescriber experiences countertransference unease

use of medications is unnecessarily interfering with their personal agency and further growth (e.g., a patient who takes an as-needed drug for almost any bad feeling, however reasonable that feeling is). As noted in Chapter 6, prescribers may become aware of the problem through a countertransference sense of unease about their patients' condition or medication use or through feelings of guilt or shame. Often, patients become attached to medications that are experienced as helpful (although countertherapeutic use may also involve being harmed by medication). Prescribers may feel pressure to prescribe more despite their internal resistance. They may also become aware of ways that patients are attached to diagnoses associated with medications, using the diagnosis to justify unhealthy behaviors or choices or to defer personal responsibility for the illness or treatment.

Addressing Countertherapeutic Uses of Medications

Given that countertherapeutic use of medication or treatment serves important but frequently unconscious purposes, patients may not be highly motivated to question this use. The ability to do so is served by having established a strong (or as strong as possible) therapeutic alliance in which it is understood that deeper questions will be raised and that the patient (and prescriber) cannot be seen as fully conscious of all motivations underlying treatment seeking.

Frame the Treatment Agreement Around Health Rather Than Absence of Symptoms

What is "countertherapeutic" may hinge on the nature of the alliance and the identified tasks of treatment. When the initial treatment agreement includes a focus not only on symptomatic relief but also on development, it may be easier to identify uses of medications that relieve symptoms while also interfering with development or promoting chronification (Isler 1988) of illness.

Some countertherapeutic effects can be anticipated and addressed specifically in the negotiation of a treatment agreement, such as when a patient has demonstrated a clear pattern of developmentally harmful medication use or when ingrained character defenses (e.g., narcissistic, obsessive, and histrionic) have been temporarily disabled by a depressive episode (Marcus 1990). For instance, a person with depleted narcissism who is in the midst of a depressive episode may experience the emptiness, superficiality, and desperation that are integral to the narcissistic solution. In this state, the patient feels motivated to change and is most likely to seek and earnestly engage in psychotherapy. Successful antidepressant treatment, however, can easily allow that patient to restore grandiose defenses, obscuring the narcissistic plight for which the patient originally sought treatment. In such cases, the pharmacotherapist may discuss with the patient (and the patient's therapist, if different from the prescriber) the potential for antidepressants to undercut the patient's readiness to change. The patient may work to hold onto depressive insights even as the depression resolves.

Although prescribers may be tempted to withhold or discontinue medications that could undermine motivation to change in such situations, this decision should be shared with patients, with as fully informed consent as possible about the potential risks. For prescribers to decide unilaterally not to offer treatment is, as Cabaniss (2001) noted, "analogous to withholding cholesterol lowering medication from a group of hypercholesterolemic diabetics who are noncompliant with dietary restrictions for fear that effective medications will eliminate their motivation for dietary control" (p. 165). Generally, except in situations in which patients are (mis)using medications in ways that are potentially toxic, harm to patients that derives from the level of meaning rarely requires immediate medication discontinuation.

Optimally, when harm from medications is mediated by meaning, it can be addressed at the level of meaning. For example, when patients undermine their own agency in the way they defensively strip feelings of meaning or attempt to blame medications (or their limitations) for untoward consequences of their own choices or lifestyles, prescribers should consistently question how the patient knows the medication is to blame, given the complicated interactions of meaning and biology. If a strong enough alliance has developed, and the prescriber has a clear idea about the patient's misuses of medications, this may be directly interpreted to the patient.

Mr. U is a middle-aged man with a personality disorder and a history of suicide attempts who seeks treatment in a psychodynamic residential program for unremitting depression with anxious distress. Mr. U is in a split treatment, with psychotherapy four times a week from one provider and psychopharmacology from another. His selective serotonin reuptake inhibitor has been replaced with a serotonin-norepinephrine reuptake inhibitor, and he is in discussion with his prescriber about tapering off of his low-dosage benzodiazepine. However, as he progresses in the treatment, his panic attacks return, requiring larger dosages of as-needed anxiolytics. The dosage increase helps for no more than a few days before his anxiety escalates again. When his prescriber attempts to explore the precipitants of his panic, Mr. U is unaware of any reason for his anxiety. Ultimately, the psychopharmacologist tells the patient that he will prescribe no more anxiolytics, instructing Mr. U to call when he is having a panic attack so that they might meet and attempt to understand what precisely the medication is meant to treat.

In the urgently scheduled meeting that follows the next time Mr. U has a panic attack, the context of his panic comes into focus. In this case (and many others, it soon becomes apparent), he left therapy in a state of quiet rage, having wanted some overt sign of caring or comfort from his therapist. He was angry both at his therapist for depriving him of a simple gesture of love and at himself for needing it. As he returned to his room, his thoughts turned to suicide, and he began forming a plan. The thought of dying, however, made him extremely anxious, precipitating a panic attack. On inquiry, the patient observes that his anxiety commonly emerges after psychotherapy hours and that he has not told the therapist of his frustration or anger. The psychopharmacologist reflects back to the patient that he appears to be requesting anxiolytics so that he can plan his suicide without anxiety, which hardly seems like an appropriate use of medications. The patient agrees to discuss his anger with the therapist. Mr. U, his therapist, and the psychopharmacologist meet together to review the dynamic in which the negative transference has been split out, "biologized," and left to the psychopharmacologist to detoxify. They agree that further anxiolytics are not warranted at this time. The patient's "treatment-resistant" anxiety remits when the negative transference is identified and engaged in the therapy.

Explore How Problems in the Alliance May Contribute to Misuse of Medications

Prescribers may also leverage the alliance in addressing patients' countertherapeutic use of medications. When medications are used in ways that contravene the agreement to use medications in support of growth, the prescriber can notice that the patient appears unilaterally to have changed the terms of the treatment agreement and wonder why he or she has given up working straightforwardly with the doctor. Exploring how a misalliance has emerged may help reestablish the alliance. Prescribers should also consider how they may have contributed to problems in the alliance. Furthermore, patients' misuse of medications can demonstrate the deleterious interpersonal consequences of such behavior because the behavior has put the doctor–patient relationship on tenuous footing.

Support Healthy Strategies to Replace Countertherapeutic Uses of Medications

When developmental harm has occurred and a patient has developed actual deficits (e.g., a real lack of coping skills, as opposed to an idea of the self as defective), psychosocial remediation should be a part of the treatment plan (e.g., long-term psychodynamic psychotherapy or dialectical behavior therapy to help the patient learn to better manage painful affects). The treatment agreement might also include limiting medications, by decreasing either absolute numbers or the availability of pills, to increase opportunities for developing affect competence. In a residential treatment setting, for example, a patient who is normally responsible for self-administering her medications may establish a plan to talk to someone first when she is in a state of emotional distress, only gaining access to as-needed medications after trying to contain her feelings with interpersonal support from nurses or counselors.

Set Limits

When the patient's countertherapeutic use of medications proves too gratifying, and insight, leveraging the alliance, and other efforts do not interrupt the misuse, the prescriber need not feel compelled to collude with the patient's demands. When it becomes a question of conscience, medication discontinuation is crucial to maintaining the integrity of the doctor–patient relationship. The pharmacotherapist may negotiate discontinuation of the medication or, if the patient's countertherapeutic use is dangerous or entrenched enough, may make discontinuation of the medication a condition of continuing pharmacological treatment. When a valued medication is threatened, some patients will be motivated to seek another treatment. If the provider has been able to cultivate a strong alliance, the patient will face a true dilemma in choosing between the doctor and the drug. Such was the case with Ms. J (Chapter 6), whose use of medications, although helpful for her anxiety, contributed in several ways to adverse outcomes. Her pursuit of complete anxiolysis dulled appropriate negative affects that would alert healthier persons that their behaviors were destructive. Moreover, her defensive attachment to her diagnosis ("It's not my fault, it's my bipolar") split her negative characteristics into her illness, making it the doctor's job to manage and giving her worst impulses free rein.

> Ms. J's psychiatrist is immediately aware that her attachment to her diagnosis is defensive and that her use of medications seems to undermine her affect competence. Although his initial impulse to set a firm limit from the outset of treatment may save him some challenging work ahead, he chooses instead to tolerate her irrational use of medications for a time while he works on es-

tablishing an alliance. From the outset, however, he expresses his own questions about her diagnosis, given his understanding of how complicated the relationship is between mind and body. Fairly quickly, he asks her to see a therapist whom he trusts while he begins, empathically, to talk with her about the grief, guilt, and other bad feelings that she is trying to eliminate. Within a few months of once-monthly meetings, in which he frames the treatment in terms of Ms. J's developmental goals, he revises the diagnosis to borderline personality disorder and begins interpreting the ways her medications have likely contributed to the losses in her life. Shortly after, he informs her that in accordance with the dictate to "do no harm," he can no longer, in good conscience, continue dulling her with a suppressant regimen and announces a plan to taper her off of gabapentin. This strains the relationship, and Ms. J not only protests vociferously but also threatens to leave treatment. The psychiatrist's empathic understanding of her losses and his clear intention to get her stable and in control enough that she can regain custody of her daughter keeps her in treatment.

Although patients may choose to leave treatment, this does not necessarily indicate a failure in or of the work. In fact, holding a critical limit with patients can be an important clinical intervention. If prescribers thoughtfully lay out and interpret an integrated understanding of patients' antidevelopmental and countertherapeutic uses of a particular medication, this may serve to highlight, in the here and now, the ways that the patients' attachment to their medications interferes with other important aspects of their lives. This includes treatment aimed at helping them achieve their developmental goals. Furthermore, if an integrated understanding of the antidevelopmental and countertherapeutic uses of a medication can be offered to the next prescriber, destructive attachments to medications, including the destruction of the previous treatment relationship, can be engaged early in subsequent treatments. In the end, it is preferable to give no treatment than to provide treatment that does more harm than good.

Key Points

- Countertransference unease may be a clue as to the presence of significant treatment resistance *from* medications.

- Identifying and addressing meaning-based iatrogenic effects and antidevelopmental uses of medications is a possible alternative to medication discontinuation.

- Real developmental deficits resulting from long-standing countertherapeutic use of medications may require remediation and not just insight into the problem.

- Prescribers should consider how countertherapeutic use of medications reflects problems in the therapeutic alliance and how they contribute to those problems.

- Unilateral prescribing decisions to discontinue medication may be necessary when countertherapeutic uses are more rewarding to the patient than growth or clinical improvement.

References

Cabaniss DL: Beyond dualism: psychoanalysis and medication in the 21st century. Bull Menninger Clin 65(2):160–170, 2001 11407140

Isler H: Headache drugs provoking chronic headache: historical aspects and common misunderstandings, in Drug-Induced Headache: Advances in Applied Neurological Sciences, Vol 5. Edited by Diener HC, Wilkinson M. New York, Springer, 1988, pp 87–94

Marcus ER: Integrating psychopharmacotherapy, psychotherapy, and mental structure in the treatment of patients with personality disorders and depression. Psychiatr Clin North Am 13(2):255–263, 1990 2191280

Identify, Contain, and Use Countertransference

The working distresses of psychiatrists are rarely fully conscious or owned openly, and (almost) never discussed as facts which merit scientific study. Rather they are suppressed, even repressed, as something we must rise above, something professionally shameful; subjectivity as a primary fact is rarely studied or valued because it is a menace to the idealized defence of objectivity. The doctor's strains are not however abolished by silence, merely hidden, and like the return of the repressed in neurosis they return in disguised forms, like pirates, sailing under flags of false objectivity and spurious science.

—Tom Main, "Traditional Psychiatric Defences
Against Close Encounter With Patients" (1977)

Prescribers may contribute to treatment resistance when they introduce unimpeded irrational processes into the prescribing process. The containment of irrationality is why pharmacotherapy strives to ground itself in evidence. Psychiatric prescribers, however, often do not work in accordance with the best available evidence (Vijapura et al. 2016). Although the evidence offers guidance not only about what to prescribe but also how to prescribe, the latter is often neglected, leaving prescribers to act out their own predilections. Even with diligent attention to the evidence base, prescribers are almost always working at the edges of the evidence because real patients do not fit the mold provided by it, requiring more creative solutions.

From a psychodynamic perspective, prescribers are as likely (or nearly as likely) as patients to be influenced by factors that are not rational. Although understanding that patients are complex systems in which subjective experience plays a major role, prescribers may work in systems that induce them to experience patients in irrationally reductive ways. Stress may also push prescribers self-protectively to think in overly simplistic ways (Bar-Tal et al.

147

2013). Patients who are overflowing with distressing feelings often evoke related feelings in their caregivers. Prescribers, in turn, may fall back on familiar defenses (Main 1977, 1978) and may prescribe in order to be rid of these feelings (e.g., prescribing a sedating regimen to an energetically demanding patient who provokes feelings of inadequacy and being overwhelmed). Evidence suggests that medical decision making is dominated by irrational factors when working with patients who are difficult to treat (Waldinger and Frank 1989).

Because it is aimed at relieving prescribers' distress, countertransference prescribing is less likely to address patients' needs. Furthermore, it is a form of misalliance that can impair the working relationship. Patients who are sensitive to their doctor's needs may respond to such medication with a masochistic surrender that impairs their authority, or it may spark their resistance and lead to power struggles in the relationship.

Learn to Recognize Countertransference

Managing countertransference in prescribing begins with recognizing that it is happening. In addition to understanding how external factors affect their ability to think more fully, prescribers should also cultivate an awareness of personal valences that may easily interact with those of their patients or systems of treatment. Does the doctor need to be liked? To feel respected, helpful, or in control? To do no harm? To be seen as caring or tolerant? To never lose hope? To the extent that prescribers are aware of the interpersonal positions in which their defenses are most likely to be activated, they will be able to recognize and thoughtfully manage difficult countertransferences more easily. Such was the case for Dr. Q (see Chapter 8), who had to learn to step back to gain perspective when gripped by the fear that he might have caused harm.

Strong feelings evoked by patients, either positive or negative, are an obvious signal to pause and consider whether one's medical judgment is affected by countertransference. Without this awareness, atypical dosages and complex or irrational medication regimens may develop and can serve as another indicator of countertransference-driven prescribing. When patients, particularly those who rely on primitive defenses, evoke strong feelings and defensive reactions in their prescribers, this is often accompanied by feelings of shame or guilt and persecutory anxieties (Shapiro and Carr 1993). The feeling that one wants to hide one's work should serve as a signal that consultation with a colleague may be helpful. Just as patients' requests for medication changes should alert doctors to consider transference aspects, when doctors contemplate making changes in treatment, they might usefully consider whether their motivation for doing so stems from countertransference (Busch and Auchincloss 1995). Moreover, referring patients for psychotherapy, consultation, or other adjunctive treatments, although often helpful for these patients, may also signal a prescriber's unconscious wish to be rid of the patient (Busch and Auchincloss 1995) and indicate a need for the prescriber to contemplate his or her unconscious motivations.

Turn Countertransference From an Impediment Into a Tool

In cases in which a patient's dysphoria is infectious, provoking intense feelings of anger, hopelessness, helplessness, or even despair in the prescriber, one path is to prescribe medications with the unconscious aim of decreasing these feelings. On the other hand, countertransference-driven impulses to prescribe can become valuable sources of data about patients' experience and inner life. To the extent that these countertransferences are transmitted through projective identification and concordant (Racker 1957) with some aspect of the patients' emotional experience, they may become a source of empathy and serve to fortify the treatment alliance. As one psychiatrist put it: "I was quite frustrated by the way she made me feel so helpless, but then I realized that that was the feeling that she lived with almost every minute of every day." When bad feelings are recontextualized as serving a useful end, and prescribers come to understand that they are not just suffering *because of* these patients but *on behalf of* them (or their treatment), these feelings may become much easier to bear.

Consult With Colleagues

The issue of countertransference emphasizes the importance of consulting with colleagues when working with patients who are difficult to treat. Such patients often cannot be treated in isolation and can push average prescribers to the limits of their pharmacological knowledge, creativity, and emotions. Colleagues who are at a distance from the transference-countertransference tangle can function as a necessary "third" (Muller 1999, 2007), offering perspective on rational prescribing while also helping the prescriber recognize and contain intense feelings evoked in the doctor–patient dyad. Systems are in no way immune to prescribing enactments in the face of strong feelings (Swenson and Wood 1990), however, and in more difficult cases, it may be useful to seek consultation from someone who has greater distance from the clinical case and who is outside of the treatment system in question.

Role of the Psychodynamic Formulation

Chapter 9 highlighted the importance of the psychodynamic formulation as a guide for understanding predominant dynamics operating in patients that could potentially impact the usefulness of pharmacotherapy. This formulation, or overall diagnosis, has other important uses as well. In particular, it may help prescribers manage unhelpful countertransference reactions. It can exert a containing and conservative effect, orienting prescribers and others under the pressure of strong or disorganizing affects. A self-aware prescriber with a formulation of repetitive patterns in the patient's life is more likely to anticipate prescribing enactments (e.g., when the prescriber re-creates the dynamic of a parent who cannot tolerate the strong affects of her child).

A dynamic formulation has also been shown to help providers maintain empathy toward challenging patients (Treloar 2009). Such was the case in the treatment of Ms. F (see Chapter 5). The patient's seeming attempts to fight her prescriber's best efforts left the prescriber feeling frustrated and helpless. Although initially the prescriber fought these feelings by prescribing more aggressively, he came to understand the unconscious logic of Ms. F's resistance. If her antipsychotic regimen were to succeed, she would be faced with the unbearable loss of her child. Understanding what the patient was facing restored the prescriber's empathy and allowed him to prescribe less aggressively while the patient worked on grief issues in her therapy. Eventually, with time and space to address the sources of her resistance, she was able to tolerate a transition to clozapine, with an overall good outcome.

A dynamic formulation need not be a thousand-word document. A brief and focused formulation of their patients' relationship to medications and treaters is generally sufficient for prescribers. Such a formulation might, for example, help predict that a patient with deep-seated issues around control might attempt to wrest control of the medications from the doctor or that a patient who could neither bear nor articulate a desperate feeling of helplessness may powerfully evoke that same feeling in the treater. When in the thrall of strong countertransference feelings, prescribers can call on the formulation, which can serve as a clinical compass that allows them to identify and contain potential irrational processes in the pharmacotherapeutic relationship so the treatment can be steered in a more thoughtful direction.

Similarly, a dynamic formulation that contains a systems perspective, if shared, can help prescribers contain irrational processes in the larger treatment system. If this works well, prescribers will benefit from only having to deal with uncontained irrationality on one front: their patient. Including the brief dynamic formulation in the patient's chart is a way to pass on accumulated wisdom about that patient and to inoculate future providers from predictable enactments.

Key Points

- Prescribers may contribute to treatment resistance when they introduce irrational processes into treatment.

- Countertransference prescribing may be contained when prescribers learn their unique countertransference tendencies and learn to identify signs of countertransference.

- Countertransference may be used as a tool for understanding patients and developing empathy.

- Consulting with colleagues is important when working with patients who are difficult to treat.

- A psychodynamic formulation may help preserve empathy when working with challenging patients.

References

Bar-Tal Y, Shrira A, Keinan G: The effect of stress on cognitive structuring: a cognitive motivational model. Pers Soc Psychol Rev 17(1):87–99, 2013 23070219

Busch FN, Auchincloss EL: The psychology of prescribing and taking medication, in Psychodynamic Concepts in General Psychiatry. Edited by Schwartz H, Bleiberg E, Weissman S. Washington, DC, American Psychiatric Press, 1995, pp 401–416

Main TF: Traditional psychiatric defences against close encounter with patients. Can Psychiatr Assoc J 22(8):457–466, 1977 597809

Main TF: Some medical defences against involvement with patients. Journal of the Balint Society 6:3–11, 1978

Muller JP: Consultation from the position of the third. Am J Psychoanal 59(2):113–118, 1999 10407636

Muller JP: A view from Riggs: treatment resistance and patient authority-IV: why the pair needs the third. J Am Acad Psychoanal Dyn Psychiatry 35(2):221–241, 2007 17650976

Racker H: The meanings and uses of countertransference. Psychoanal Q 26(3):303–357, 1957 13465913

Shapiro ER, Carr AW: Lost in Familiar Places: Creating New Connections Between the Individual and Society. New Haven, CT, Yale University Press, 1993

Swenson CR, Wood MJ: Issues involved in combining drugs with psychotherapy for the borderline inpatient. Psychiatr Clin North Am 13(2):297–306, 1990 2352892

Treloar AJ: Effectiveness of education programs in changing clinicians' attitudes toward treating borderline personality disorder. Psychiatr Serv 60(8):1128–1131, 2009 19648203

Vijapura S, Laferton JA, Mintz D, et al: Psychiatrists' attitudes toward nonpharmacologic factors within the context of antidepressant pharmacotherapy. Acad Psychiatry 40(5):783–789, 2016 26646406
Waldinger RJ, Frank AF: Clinicians' experiences in combining medication and psychotherapy in the treatment of borderline patients. Hosp Community Psychiatry
40(7):712–718, 1989 2777227

• CHAPTER 14 •

Who Is Psychodynamic Psychopharmacology For?

Patient Characteristics

We are all more simply human than otherwise.

—Harry Stack Sullivan

The core principles of psychodynamic psychopharmacology were developed from work with a diagnostically heterogeneous group of patients for whom the common element was a history of treatment resistance. Accordingly, the theory and technique of psychodynamic psychopharmacology are not focused on any particular diagnostic category but rather on the kinds of real-world patients with complex comorbidities who are often referred for specialized psychiatric evaluation and treatment, having failed both first- and second-line approaches (Table 14–1).

Given that character disorders and immature defenses are commonly correlated with treatment resistance, many of the patients for whom psychodynamic psychopharmacology is most helpful are those whose character pathology interferes with healthy use of medications. This may take the form of rigid defenses that are fortified by symptoms (see Chapter 5) or by medications (see Chapter 6) or of pronounced negative transferences (conscious or unconscious) that interfere with patients' ability to utilize prescribers' treatment recommendations.

Character disorders are not the only conditions that interfere with pharmacotherapy. Significant social problems may also complicate patients' response to medications when problems of living are conflated with problems of illness and when secondary gains change the hedonic calculus for these

Table 14–1. Optimal patient characteristics for psychodynamic
             psychopharmacology

Ability to enter into a therapeutic alliance

Ability, with help, to reflect on self and relationship to pharmacotherapy

Ambivalent motivation to change

Complex transferences to caregiving

Pharmacological treatment resistance

Psychological factors that interfere with agency in relation to illness and medications

Some secondary benefit derived from symptoms or the sick role

patients. Severe anxiety can lead to rigid overreliance on defenses that impede the intended effects of medications. Trauma, social disempowerment,
and other adverse childhood experiences may also promote hypertrophied
defenses and the negative expectations of caregiving that feed into treatment
resistance. Patients with psychosis may also benefit from psychodynamic
psychopharmacology as long as they retain a degree of observing ego.

Limitations of Psychodynamic
Psychopharmacology

As a clinical approach, psychodynamic psychopharmacology makes particular demands on patients to be active agents in their own recovery. The authority and responsibility extended to patients are not optimal for everyone.
The model presumes that, although ambivalent about aspects of pharmacotherapy, patients ultimately want to benefit from treatment. Patients who ultimately are not motivated to use medications in healthy ways are unlikely to
make use of their agency in treatment. An example is the patients with soci-
opathy whose main interest in seeking care is to procure substances of abuse
under the guise of treatment. Of course, with such patients, it may take time
to learn that they are essentially unambivalent about using medications in
countertherapeutic ways.

   Psychodynamic psychopharmacology also presumes patients will be able
and willing to reflect on their relationship with pharmacotherapy, to consider unconscious aspects of their experience of medications and treatment,
and to work on problems in the pharmacotherapeutic alliance. Conditions
that interfere with reflective functioning will restrict the capacity to make use
of psychodynamic psychopharmacology. Severe intellectual disability and
significant neurocognitive disorders limit patients' ability to develop their
agency, reflect on sources of treatment resistance, and learn from experience
in the context of the therapeutic relationship.

Severe psychotic illness and acute affective psychoses are also a relative contraindication to the unmodified use of psychodynamic psychopharmacology. Patients with less severe psychosis who have retained capacity for an observing ego may benefit significantly from this model, which does not presume that either patient or doctor is the arbiter of reality but rather posits that learning is an important task of the pharmacotherapeutic alliance. More severe psychosis, however, may impair patients' capacity to reflect on experience, reality test, and effectively engage as partners in the pharmacotherapeutic alliance. When patients are stabilized, the work of psychodynamic psychopharmacology may address dynamics that could lead to psychotic relapse, such as by exploring the soundness of psychotic beliefs that lead to nonadherence (e.g., the magical wish that not taking antipsychotics would mean that one was not psychotic) or questioning a patient's deauthorizing assumptions that support passivity and therapeutic pessimism.

Adaptation of Psychodynamic Psychopharmacology

Although full application of the techniques of psychodynamic psychopharmacology may not be appropriate for all patients, most treatments can benefit from modified or partial implementation, as guided by clinical judgment.

Severe Impairments in Mental Functioning

Patients with a significant intellectual disability may not have the capacity to join prescribers in making informed decisions about medications based on developmental goals, reflect on their relationship with medications, and address issues in the pharmacotherapeutic alliance. However, it may still benefit treatment for prescribers to develop an integrated, psychodynamically informed, biopsychosocial understanding of the patients' wishes for treatment and sources of potential resistance based on an understanding of the patients' history and psychology. Treatment can then be modulated based on those understandings.

Similarly, regardless of patients' intellectual and reality testing capacities, treatment is likely to benefit from attention to the pharmacotherapeutic alliance, including the evidence-based factors described in Chapter 2, such as empathy, warmth, and interest in the patients' recovery. In this case, prescribers should also be aware of potential misuses of medications, whether by the patients or the treatment system in which they are embedded. In cases of impaired agency, prescribers must consider their own participation in irrational processes, given that patients may not be in a position to challenge prescribers' irrational use of medications.

Treatment-Naïve and Treatment-Responsive Conditions

Although the principles of psychodynamic psychopharmacology were developed to address the treatment needs of patients who have not responded to multiple treatments, most of these techniques can also benefit patients who are treatment naïve and may further enhance outcomes in patients who are treatment responsive. An extensive evidence base (see Chapter 2) suggests that a nonreductionistic, patient-centered approach that considers patients' developmental goals, attends to their anxieties and ambivalences, focuses on maintaining a solid alliance, involves them in decision making, and calls on prescribers to be self-reflective is likely to contribute positively to outcomes in any treatment.

For treatment-naïve patients, there would be little call, for example, to address countertherapeutic uses of medications. At the same time, the psychodynamic psychopharmacologist would be in a position to identify, early on, beliefs and attitudes about illness and medications that could promote psychiatric chronification (Isler 1988) and to address these issues before they lead to treatment resistance. For example, when a patient understands the prescription of a medication to imply a purely biogenic theory of illness, it can lead to prognostic pessimism and decreased mood-regulation expectancies (Kemp et al. 2014). The prescriber would be in a position to identify this and address it through psychoeducation and possibly also by interpreting the underlying dynamics promoting a reductionistic view.

For treatment-resistant patients, it is reasonable not to assign too much potency to pharmacotherapy. Overly optimistic assessments run the risk of promoting passivity that undermines treatment. Furthermore, patients who have failed previous trials do not generally prefer prescribers to be too optimistic (Priebe et al. 2017) because this is discordant with their experience. With treatment-naïve patients, however, there may be reason to raise expectations for an initial treatment, given the significant impact of the placebo effect and treatment expectancies. The task of prescribers in such cases is to raise expectancies without undermining patient authority (e.g., by discussing how the patient's expectancies could contribute to a robust response). In both treatment-naïve and treatment-resistant populations, it is helpful to emphasize that patients play an important role in their own recovery.

Treatment-Resistant Medical Conditions

In keeping with the pioneering work of Michael Balint (1957) and contemporary research on the value of patient-centered approaches (Stewart et al. 2000), it appears that the techniques of psychodynamic psychopharmacology can also be applied effectively to chronic and treatment-resistant medical conditions. Particularly when medical treatment has been complicated by patient nonadherence with recommendations, lack of follow-up, nocebo responsiveness, overutilization of treatment, poor therapeutic alliance, and impaired functioning that goes beyond the degree of symptomatic distress, modified techniques may prove extremely useful. The applications of psychodynamic psychopharmacology for chronic medical conditions in integrated care are explored further in Chapter 19.

Key Points

- The principles of psychodynamic psychopharmacology were designed specifically for enhancing the outcomes of treatment-refractory psychiatric patients.

- These principles can also be helpful in working with treatment-resistant medical patients and psychiatric patients who are not treatment refractory.

- These techniques are limited in patients with serious cognitive impairments, major impairments in reality testing, major difficulties forming a therapeutic alliance, or a true lack of interest in recovery.

References

Balint M: The Doctor and His Patient and the Illness. London, Pitman, 1957

Isler H: Headache drugs provoking chronic headache: historical aspects and common misunderstandings, in Drug-Induced Headache. (Advances in Applied Neurological Sciences, Vol 5. Edited by Diener HC, Wilkinson M.) New York, Springer, 1988, pp 87–94

Kemp JJ, Lickel JJ, Deacon BJ: Effects of a chemical imbalance causal explanation on individuals' perceptions of their depressive symptoms. Behav Res Ther 56:47–52, 2014 24657311

Priebe S, Ramjaun G, Strappelli N, et al: Do patients prefer optimistic or cautious psychiatrists? An experimental study with new and long-term patients. BMC Psychiatry 17(1):26, 2017 28095888

Stewart M, Brown JB, Donner A, et al: The impact of patient-centered care on outcomes. J Fam Pract 49(9):796–804, 2000 11032203

• CHAPTER 15 •

Before Initiating Treatment

He who is best prepared can best serve his moment of inspiration.

—Samuel Taylor Coleridge

Psychodynamic psychopharmacology marries time-honored psychodynamic insights with an evidence base that connects meaning factors to medication response. Successful practice of this approach is grounded in a set of knowledge, skills, and attitudes that supports the effective use of its specific techniques. These domains (Figure 15–1) include 1) having a basic grasp of the evidence base that connects meaning and medication, 2) having a basic grasp of psychodynamic theory and technique, and 3) developing specific clinical virtues that facilitate a psychologically attuned and nonauthoritarian approach to patients. It is also helpful for practitioners to be attuned to covert pressures in the treatment environment that potentially undercut the ability to use the techniques of psychodynamic psychopharmacology.

Become Familiar With the Evidence Bases

A central component of psychodynamic psychopharmacology is the ability to integrate the evidence bases that guide *what* to prescribe and *how* to prescribe. Part of the work of forging an alliance with patients involves conveying relevant knowledge from this evidence base to help establish a therapeutic rationale for this way of working and to help patients appreciate their potential role in optimizing treatment outcomes. Thus, prescribers must understand the evidence base well enough to convey it and to develop an alliance around it. Chapter 2 provided a basis for understanding how key psychological and interpersonal factors may shape the outcome of pharmacotherapy for psychiatric distress, and this should be adequate for beginning practitioners, although it can certainly be useful to supplement with other reviews (Greenberg 2016; Mintz and Flynn 2012).

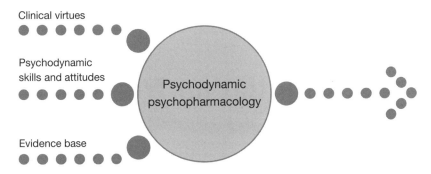

Figure 15–1.   Preparatory elements of psychodynamic psychopharma-
                cology.

Ideally, by understanding the import of psychological and social/interpersonal factors in pharmacotherapy, practitioners of psychodynamic psychopharmacology will seek continuing education in this area of psychiatric care. Indeed, after a quarter-century of biomedical reductionism, the field of psychiatry is rediscovering the psychosocial dimension of care, and relevant research is being published monthly. For example, keeping attuned to research on placebo and nocebo effects; the therapeutic alliance in pharmacotherapy; the role of patient preferences, expectations, and activation for treatment outcome; patient-centeredness; and related factors will ensure that practitioners are guided by up-to-date evidence.

Given that providers of continuing medical education (in psychiatry, at least) have not necessarily caught up with these emerging developments in psychiatric prescribing, it can be helpful for practitioners to request more education about this aspect of the evidence base.

Apply Psychodynamic Thinking

The practice of psychodynamic psychopharmacology requires that practitioners have a basic level of understanding and skill. Psychiatrists who have completed training in Accreditation Council for Graduate Medical Education–accredited residencies may possess these basic skills in general, most having achieved the level of "competency" in psychodynamic psychotherapy during residency training. With these skills, psychiatric prescribers should be able to appreciate the impact of unconscious and nonconscious factors on patients' behavior, the extent to which patients (and doctors) are roiled by internal conflicts regarding treatment and health, and the potential potency of transference effects. Furthermore, psychiatric prescribers will have developed at least rudimentary skills in providing interpretations of unconscious content that interferes with treatment.

What these psychodynamically trained providers were likely not taught is an integrative way of thinking about medications as simultaneously biologically and symbolically active. Chapter 3 offers such a framework for considering how a psychodynamically informed approach to prescribing may be conducted. Similarly, Chapters 4 through 7 provide a basis for understanding some of the basic psychodynamics of pharmacological treatment resistance. An understanding of the common dynamics of such resistance helps address the mind-body and psychotherapy-psychopharmacology split that is often conveyed as part of the "hidden curriculum" in psychiatry education. Together, these chapters are a prerequisite for psychodynamically trained psychiatrists to practice psychodynamic psychopharmacology.

Other psychiatric prescribers, including primary care providers, physician assistants, and nurse practitioners, will likely not have received specific or extensive training in psychodynamic psychotherapy. As such, they may require additional training in the application of psychodynamic concepts and techniques. Further training in psychodynamic psychopharmacology is one path to developing competence. Balint groups (Adams et al. 2006; Balint 1957), in which medical care providers work together with a trained group leader to process the psychological aspects of caring for difficult-to-treat patients, offer another path to developing competence in psychodynamic formulations and techniques. Such groups are common in many primary care residencies and are available in many clinical communities for those seeking to develop a deeper understanding of the doctor–patient relationship and of psychological factors involved in treatment resistance.

Develop Clinical Virtues

Even before the question of what to do, there is the question of who to be (Radden and Sadler 2008, 2010). Psychodynamic virtues (Brenner and Khan 2013) grounded in prescribers' fundamental capacities support the development of respectful prescriber–patient relationships and offer prescribers internal guidance about technical approaches to their patients.

Perhaps foremost among the clinical virtues that support the practice of psychodynamic psychopharmacology is *psychological-mindedness* (Appelbaum 1973), or *reflective functioning* (Fonagy et al. 1998). This refers to the mental capacity to reflect on the minds of others as well as one's own (Lingiardi and McWilliams 2017), to be able to differentiate ideas and feelings from reality, and to consider the symbolic meaning of behavior. Reflective capacities, although often developed prior to becoming a psychiatric provider, can be cultivated through the use of personal psychotherapy (Allen and Fonagy 2006; Björgvinsson and Hart 2006) and other techniques (Parker and Leggett 2012; Shoenberg and Yakeley 2014; Yakeley et al. 2011).

Awareness of the complexity introduced by unconscious psychological processes for both prescribers and patients paves the way for other virtues, such as empathy, curiosity, humility, nondefensiveness, tolerance for ambiguity, and a nonauthoritarian approach to the doctor–patient relationship. Empathy may be deepened by recognizing that the patient and prescriber are far more alike than different, both being shaped by deep, often primitive, unconscious processes. Curiosity is raised by the awareness that there is almost always more going on than meets the eye. Awareness that prescribers are blinded to their own conflicts may make it easier for them nondefensively to ask, "How is the patient right?" (Shapiro 2019). Furthermore, true recognition of the complicating role of psychological processes necessitates both a therapeutic humility about the limits of prescribers' understanding and a tolerance of ambiguity.

Attend to Reductionistic Pressures

As described in Chapters 7 and 13, prescribers often face significant pressure, both from the systems in which they work and from their own psychology, to think reductionistically about their patients and about prescribing. Becoming aware of their own sensitivities and countertransference proclivities supports prescribers' capacity to identify and contain these pressures. Of course, their individual psychotherapy is one such place in which particular transference-countertransference valences can be identified. It can also be useful to develop peer support networks to assist with identifying such internal and external pressures and to find support in resisting them. Balint groups are one formalized approach to identifying these pressures, but more informal peer networks of like-minded prescribers are also beneficial. Too often, prescribers believe they are alone in valuing the human dimension of pharmacotherapy, especially when they operate within a system that eclipses spaces for reflection and encourages a biomedical-pharmacological approach to patients.

Prescribers who have obtained basic training in psychodynamics, mastered the evidence base for the psychosocial dimension of pharmacotherapy, and developed psychodynamic virtues, such as psychological-mindedness, empathy, and humility, should have the tools to apply the principles and techniques of psychodynamic psychopharmacology.

Key Points

- To optimize pharmacotherapy outcomes, prescribers should be familiar not only with evidence bases regarding effective medications but also with elements of effective prescribing processes.

- Psychological-mindedness, empathy, curiosity, therapeutic humility, and tolerance for ambiguity are clinical virtues that can be developed and that support the effective use of psychodynamic psychopharmacology.

- Maintaining an integrated perspective in psychodynamic psychopharmacology may be optimized by an awareness of intrapsychic, interpersonal, and systemic pressures to think reductionistically.

References

Adams KE, O'Reilly M, Romm J, et al: Effect of Balint training on resident professionalism. Am J Obstet Gynecol 195(5):1431–1437, 2006 16996457

Allen JG, Fonagy P (eds): The Handbook of Mentalization-Based Treatment. Hoboken, NJ, Wiley, 2006

Appelbaum SA: Psychological-mindedness: word, concept and essence. Int J Psychoanal 54(1):35–46, 1973 4724251

Balint M: The Doctor and His Patient and the Illness. Pitman, London, 1957

Björgvinsson T, Hart J: Cognitive behavioral therapy promotes mentalizing, in The Handbook of Mentalization-Based Treatment. Edited by Allen JG, Fonagy P. Hoboken, NJ, Wiley, 2006, pp 157–170

Brenner A, Khan F: The training of psychodynamic psychiatrists: the concept of "psychodynamic virtue." Psychodyn Psychiatry 41(1):57–74, 2013 23480160

Fonagy P, Target M, Steele H, et al: Reflective-Functioning Manual, Version 5.0, for Application to Adult Attachment Interviews. London, University College London, 1998

Greenberg RP: The rebirth of psychosocial importance in a drug-filled world. Am Psychol 71(8):781–791, 2016 27977264

Lingiardi V, McWilliams N (eds): Psychodynamic Diagnostic Manual: PDM-2. New York, Guilford, 2017

Mintz DL, Flynn DF: How (not what) to prescribe: nonpharmacologic aspects of psychopharmacology. Psychiatr Clin North Am 35(1):143–163, 2012 22370496

Parker S, Leggett A: Teaching the clinical encounter in psychiatry: a trial of Balint groups for medical students. Australas Psychiatry 20(4):343–347, 2012 22767937

Radden J, Sadler J: Character virtues in psychiatric practice. Harv Rev Psychiatry 16(6):373–380, 2008 19085391

Radden J, Sadler J: The Virtuous Psychiatrist: Character Ethics in Psychiatric Practice. New York, Oxford University Press, 2010

Shapiro ER: Finding a Place to Stand: Developing Self-Reflective Institutions, Leaders and Citizens. Quezon City, Philippines, Phoenix Publishing House, 2019

Shoenberg P, Yakeley J (eds): Learning About Emotions in Illness: Integrating Psychotherapeutic Teaching Into Medical Education. New York, Routledge, 2014

Yakeley J, Shoenberg P, Morris R, et al: Psychodynamic approaches to teaching medical students about the doctor-patient relationship: randomised controlled trial. The Psychiatrist 35(8):308–313, 2011

• CHAPTER 16 •

The Engagement Phase

Anyone who hopes to learn the noble game of chess from books will soon discover that only the openings and end-games admit of an exhaustive systematic presentation and that the infinite variety of moves which develop after the opening defy any such description.... The extraordinary diversity of the psychical constellations concerned, the plasticity of all mental processes and the wealth of determining factors oppose any mechanization of the technique; and they bring it about that a course of action that is as a rule justified may at times prove ineffective, whilst one that is usually mistaken may once in a while lead to the desired end. These circumstances, however, do not prevent us from laying down a procedure for the physician which is effective on the average.

—Sigmund Freud, "On Beginning the Treatment" (1913/1958)

To the extent that treatment effectiveness hinges on a solid alliance, the beginning phase of the therapeutic relationship is of paramount importance. Much of the work of psychodynamic psychopharmacology occurs within the first several hours, when crucial negotiations regarding the foundation of the treatment occur. Manifestly, these negotiations involve tasks such as beginning to form a mutual understanding of the patient's reasons for seeking treatment, psychoeducation about a biopsychosocially integrated approach to the patient's trouble, setting the treatment frame and the responsibilities of both the patient and the prescriber, and identifying dynamic factors that may interfere with optimal outcomes. More deeply, *it is the manner in which these tasks are engaged* that embodies a frame in which the patient's authority is central.

As Freud (1913/1958) noted, the first therapeutic gestures can be fairly standard because the patient's unique psychology has yet to be expressed. As such, there is limited potential in the very beginning to make specific adaptations to the patient. Psychodynamic psychopharmacologists will likely de-

165

Table 16–1. Basic tasks of the engagement phase

Establish a patient-centered alliance, focusing on developmental goals rather than symptoms

Obtain a developmental history that reveals important relational paradigms and patterns

Explore sources of ambivalence about medications, treatment, and symptoms

Assess the patient's feelings about taking medications

Express realistic humility about the limits of medications

Encourage the patient's agency in addressing psychiatric struggles

Provide psychoeducation about the impact of psychosocial factors on treatment outcome

velop their own preferred approaches for addressing the fundamental tasks of the engagement phase, as described in Table 16–1. During the engagement phase, some of the basic principles of psychodynamic psychopharmacology may be less prominent. Addressing countertherapeutic uses of medications, for example, will, in most cases, become a focus in the maintenance phase, once an alliance is established. Similarly, attending to countertransference will also become a focus later, after countertransferences have developed.

Establish a Person-Centered Focus, Including Developmental Targets

From the outset, how prescribers engage patients conveys the basic premise of this way of working—namely, that they are treating a person, not an illness. Prescribers communicate this to patients by *framing the initial questions in dimensions that are person-centered rather than illness-centered.* Practically, this means asking patients about their hopes for treatment and reframing, if necessary, a focus on symptoms into a focus on the ways that the symptoms interfere with the patients' lives (Table 16–2). A more specific focus on the nature of the symptoms can come later, as prescribers work toward diagnostic clarity. As long as patients do not *need* to focus on their symptoms, prescribers prioritize information that will contribute to the development of an overall diagnosis (Table 16–3).

> Mr. V, a 29-year-old man who is presently unemployed, presents for treatment of depression and anxiety. He was most recently prescribed lamotrigine and lurasidone at therapeutic dosages for bipolar disorder, clonazepam for anxiety, zaleplon and melatonin for insomnia, and ibuprofen three or four times daily for neck pain. He has been treated with opioids in the past but believed he was becoming dependent and detoxed himself despite ongoing

Table 16–2.   Sample developmental goals

Improved self-efficacy
Improved self-esteem
Increased capacity for enjoyment
Finding meaning
Breaking out of maladaptive patterns
Ability to succeed in school or work
Better relationships

Table 16–3.   Psychodiagnostic assessment: developing an overall diagnosis

Develop an objective-descriptive DSM diagnosis
Understand the patient's developmental goals for treatment
Understand how the patient wants to use treatment
Assess psychosocial contributions to symptoms
Understand the patient's relationship to treatment
Understand the patient's feelings about medications
Understand the patient's feelings about treatment
Understand the patient's feelings about treaters and medical authority
Assess ambivalence in the social context (e.g., family)
Assess relational schemas based on family dynamics
Identify common relational patterns
Develop a psychodynamic formulation of treatment resistance

pain. He meets with Dr. D for a 50-minute intake session for pharmacotherapy after relocating in search of a new start.

> Dr. D: I just want to begin by saying that I have a number of agendas for our first meeting. I'd like to get a sense of who you are as a person and get a basic sense of the trouble and how it impacts you. I also want to give you a sense of who I am and how I work because it might be somewhat different from what you're used to. If there's anything with your medication that needs to be changed urgently, I need to know that, too. Are there any specific agendas that you are bringing into this meeting?
> Mr. V: Um, no. Maybe I'll have something later but not right now.
> Dr. D: Then maybe we can start with why you're here, what you're hoping to get out of treatment.
> Mr. V: Well, I'm here because of my depression and my bipolar, and I have anxiety. It has really taken a toll on me. I just moved, so I need a new psychopharmacologist.

> Dr. D: I'm interested to hear some more about the toll your anxiety, depression, and bipolar symptoms have had on your life. How have they interfered with the things that are important to you?

Elicit Developmental Goals

At this juncture, the prescriber could ask about Mr. V's mood or pain symptoms, which might be typical in an illness-centered interview. Instead, she expresses interest first in his complaint of the toll his symptoms have taken. Such an approach helps maintain a person-centered focus while elucidating how the patient's symptoms have interfered with his life goals. It also demonstrates, from the outset, that Dr. D is interested in Mr. V's life and person.

> Mr. V explains how his intense emotional reactions and depressive collapses have created problems in work environments and important relationships to the point that he cannot sustain employment or friendships; he even believes his family is on the verge of giving up on him. He feels stuck in a loop that he cannot escape, and he cannot bear the idea of losing anything more. He highlights the toll these problems have had on his self-esteem and describes how he can be very critical toward himself when he encounters failure. He adds that he is probably very critical of others as well; he feels chronically let down and desperate for someone to alleviate his pain. However, people seem to abandon him when he needs them the most.
>
> Dr. D wonders about his recent move and why he is seeking treatment now. Mr. V explains that he has relocated a few hours from the rural community where he grew up and is now living with his mother and brother. He has some friends from college in the area, so he thought relocating might afford a fresh start, and seeing Dr. D was another aspect of this plan. He is also trying to decide whether to enroll in a local culinary school.

Psychodynamically Informed Biopsychosocial Assessment

Attend to Early Relational Schemas and Repeating Relational Patterns

> Listening beyond the level of Mr. V's symptoms, Dr. D notices a range of important themes that are relevant to the pharmacotherapy task. Foremost, Mr. V wishes for better social and work relationships, which may ultimately become the person-centered focus of treatment. In addition, Dr. D notices that the patient has highlighted how interpersonal conflict has become a disruptive pattern in his life and begins to consider how that pattern may play out between them, potentially interfering with aspects of pharmacotherapy. Furthermore, she recognizes how perfectionism can fuel depression and interfere with the development of a therapeutic alliance (Zuroff et al. 2000).

Suspecting that such perfectionism has deeper roots, she chooses to pick up on this theme as an entrée into the question of how Mr. V's early interpersonal experiences became a template for his subsequent relationships, presumably including the pharmacotherapy relationship.

Dr. D: It sounds like you can be very hard on yourself. Is that something you learned? Has it been that way for a long time?

Mr. V: Yeah, I had to be a perfectionist…to prove that I was good enough. My father—I call him my sperm donor—was a real jerk. He was an alcoholic, a mean one, but he hid it really well from the world and was really successful, and he singled me out because I was the one who could do something. My brother had troubles; he had autism, so I had to be the one to make up for it. I haven't talked to my dad in years, basically since he divorced my mom.

Dr. D: And how about your mom? Was she able to be a support for you?

Mr. V: Well, you know, she had my brother. He needed a lot of attention, so I don't think she was paying a lot of attention to me. She thought everything was okay with me because I was getting good grades and all.

Dr. D: You said your dad singled you out. What would he do?

Mr. V: He was always pushing me, and if I wasn't perfect, he would humiliate me. If I got a 95 on a test, he would ask what happened to the other 5 points! He would come to my games but only want to talk about the things I could do better. He would always correct me even if he didn't know what he was talking about. If I was ever good enough, he would always take the credit and say, "See, I told you to do it that way."

In this case, the patient went right from perfectionism into family dynamics. Had he not, however, Dr. D would have asked more explicitly about his early life and expressed curiosity about the impact of family patterns on his life. Given what she learned in the first 10 minutes, Dr. D noted several things that may be relevant to the prescriber–patient relationship, including issues of fairness and envy (in relation to the patient's brother), the patient's capacity to sever relationships, and most important, the fact that he could easily have a disturbed relationship with caregiving. She is alerted that the patient may be sensitive to feeling disrespected or disempowered and aware that a paternal transference (being narcissistically preoccupied, critical, and demanding) or a maternal transference (neglectfully preoccupied with other things) could represent impediments to a working alliance. More information is needed to determine which of these things might have become a pattern, so she inquires further to determine what repeating patterns might be expected to emerge in relation to the pharmacotherapy task.

Dr. D: Growing up like that can really leave a mark, like making you more perfectionistic, but I can imagine that it has affected you in a lot of different ways. Are there ways that you feel like it gets in the way of other things, of other relationships?

Mr. V: Well, I always put a lot of pressure on myself with other people. A lot of the time, I just try to avoid people because I have to try so hard, and it's exhausting, and I get upset when I don't live up to what I'm supposed to do.

Dr. D: Are you that way with other people, too? Do you expect a lot from other people as well?

Mr. V: That's the thing, I feel like I'm really tolerant, but I'm also really angry. It doesn't make sense. I do get mad, especially when my meds aren't working right, but mostly, I get mad at myself. And I get mad when people judge me, and it's unfair—well, not really mad, but frustrated.

Assess Characterological Strengths and Vulnerabilities

At this point, the prescriber has the sense that more about expectations, perfectionism, and anger will be revealed over time but reads that her patient is defensive about thinking of his own aggression or anger. She hears, also, that there may be ways he diminishes the meaning and importance of his anger by attributing it to a failure of medications, perhaps medicalizing feelings that are potentially appropriate and informative. She has begun to develop a basic sense of this patient's characterological strengths and vulnerabilities (Table 16–4) because these are likely to affect how he is able to use medications. It seems there are likely some issues around affect tolerance and tolerance of delay that are pharmacologically relevant.

> Dr. D asks Mr. V about his experiences with school and romantic relationships. He reports that college was a struggle because he got off on the wrong foot. He had had a small group of friends and binged on alcohol 3–4 days per week. His grades suffered, and his mood became more labile. After some drunken acting out at the beginning of his junior year that resulted in his being placed on disciplinary leave, he decided that he should not drink. Now, he will have a single drink a few times per year in social situations where it is called for. After he curtailed his drinking, his grades improved, but he did not find a social group and was lonely. Romantically, he has engaged in some drunken hook-ups, but at the age of 29 years, he has not yet had a serious girlfriend. When asked, he hypothesizes that self-esteem issues and fears of rejection have made him awkward around women. His mood lability persisted after he curtailed his use of alcohol, with agitation and irritability at times and periods when he fell into despair, hopelessness, and self-loathing.

The person-centered focus on the effects of illness and on basic relational paradigms has now given the prescriber a basic developmental history, enough to begin to understand both Mr. V's broader life goals (find work and love and enhance self-esteem) and the possible transferences that might adversely impact treatment. It has also begun to address other questions and to assess his ego capacities, including affect competence. In this case, it seems Mr. V is anxious about his emotional life. He gets defensive

Table 16–4. Assessing characterological strengths and vulnerabilities

Ego development	Superego development
Affect competence—can the patient use feelings?	Is the patient guided by principles?
Tolerance of delay—can the patient delay gratification?	Is it mild enough that the patient can adhere to its dictates?

when Dr. D asks questions about his feelings of anger. He seems to want to medicalize his anger and interpersonal troubles, such as when he describes his anger as emerging primarily when his medications are not working.

This process has taken almost half of the 50-minute intake session and has established that the prescriber will be paying attention to meaning and not just symptoms. At this point in the session, Dr. D turns her attention toward the symptoms and how Mr. V wants to use treatment. Given the time constraints of the initial encounter, it is not possible to fully explicate the symptoms or to achieve full diagnostic clarity. Rather, the primary aims of the initial appointment are to develop rapport and a basic assessment of the patient's symptoms. Important elements of this evaluation include how the patient understands his troubles and how he has experienced past treatment. After Dr. D has understood Mr. V better and forged a basic alliance that supports the patient's authority, follow-up sessions will be more focused on diagnostic detail and the specifics of his responses to medications. In a longer (e.g., 90-minute) intake session, Dr. D would likely achieve all of the goals of the engagement phase with this patient in one session.

> Dr. D: You've mentioned bipolar disorder, depression, and anxiety as things that have interfered with your life. I don't really understand what those things are like for you. Of all the things that are troubling you, what do you think is most important right now?

> Mr. V talks further about his depression, the accompanying lack of energy, and a desire to curl up and avoid the world. In response, Dr. D obtains more detailed information regarding the onset and frequency of Mr. V's depressive episodes and whether Mr. V has any ideas about what might provoke these episodes. The patient notes that his depression gets worse when he is under more stress, and he wonders if anxiety triggers his depression. He reports passive suicidal ideation when he is most depressed but denies active suicidality. He did once take quadruple his dose of sleeping medications but is emphatic this was an attempt to sleep and not to die. He expresses frustration that he was briefly hospitalized involuntarily after this, based on an overreaction and misunderstanding of his intent. Dr. D follows up with some questions about self-harm, and Mr. V reports that he has a history of punching himself in the head when especially frustrated.

Dr. D notices that although Mr. V describes himself as having a bipolar disorder, he has mostly talked about depression. She has questions about whether his mood lability is characterological or related to a true bipolar vulnerability. Although this differentiation is crucial to an effective treatment plan, she also hears that Mr. V feels destabilized by his anxiety. Given her understanding that anxiety serves a "signal function" in pointing toward important areas of conflict, Dr. D chooses, at this juncture, to follow up first on the sources of Mr. V's anxiety.

Dr. D: You said that anxiety and stress may trigger your depression. What's it like, your anxiety? Are there particular things that bring it on?

Mr. V: It's just anxiety, you know. I feel nervous, like something's wrong. It feels like there's too much, and I can't do it. I just kind of shut down, and I can't do anything, but I know I should do more. I feel really bad, like nervous.

Dr. D: I'm trying to understand what that looks like. Do you have an example in mind of when that happened?

Mr. V: At my last job, the owners were always saying, "You need to work harder," especially because two other people quit, and the chef was always complaining about what everyone else wasn't doing right, but he just kind of rolled in right before, and everyone else was doing extra work, stuff the chef should do also. They didn't see that I was doing the work of three people. They needed me. I kept the whole thing going. I came in at lunchtime half the time to do prep, but they kept saying "you need to be more efficient" and trying to supervise me. It was impossible. Sometimes I was in the zone, and I could get it all done, but sometimes it made me so anxious I just couldn't. It got to be too much, and I got anxious all the time, and then I started getting depressed.

Dr. D: It sounds like some of your anxiety comes from situations where it feels like someone is asking more from you than you can realistically deliver.

Mr. V: Yeah, that makes me anxious and stressed.

Dr. D: You know, some people, in a situation like that, would feel angry. Do you think you also feel angry when too much is demanded of you?

Mr. V: Not angry, I guess. Just frustrated that they won't listen, and frustrated that the chef criticizes everyone and doesn't do his part. But mostly I feel anxious and overwhelmed. I thought about quitting, and I thought I can't quit because the place will fall apart without me, but then I just got too depressed, and I had to quit.

Listen to the Meaning and Phenomenology of Symptoms

By drilling down on the phenomenology of symptoms and the patient's understanding of these symptoms, Dr. D has accomplished several things. First, she has obtained a clearer sense that narcissistic vulnerabilities likely underlie some of the patient's difficulties. Feeling disrespected or inadequate seems to be an important trigger for increased symptoms, particularly anxiety and, secondarily, depression. Although this does not rule out bipolar disorder, it is part of a picture that points toward characterological vulnerabilities that may complicate pharmacotherapy. Second, Dr. D has also listened to this material through her working hypothesis that Mr. V's mood symptoms may stem from or even guard against his substantial anger (or narcissistic rage). Furthermore, she has refined her assessment of his psychological-mindedness, language for his internal experience, affect competence, and sense of agency. It seems that, on the surface, the patient generally thinks of his symptoms in ways that are largely stripped of meaning. By asking about the constellation of events, thoughts, and feelings related to outbreaks of anxiety and impairment of functioning, she has begun to raise questions about his medicalized understanding.

Question Reductionistic Assumptions

In early sessions, it can be useful to draw attention to more complex ways of understanding patients' symptoms, reduced to neither simple biological nor psychological phenomena. In doing so, it is helpful to listen for evidence of anxiety or defensiveness that indicates where symptoms or treatment has come to serve defensive functions. In Mr. V's case, challenging more deauthorizing assumptions will mostly be left for future sessions as prescriber and patient grapple to understand the relative contribution of problems of living and problems of illness. Finally, Dr. D notes the way his father's irrationally demanding and dismissive "voice" seems to pervade Mr. V's self-concept and interpersonal relationships. For example, as Mr. V describes his recent work conflicts, he oscillates between grandiose competence (e.g., "doing the work of three people," "I kept the whole thing going") and inept collapse (e.g., "I just kind of shut down, and I can't do anything"). He then jumps to a self-critical response ("but I know I should do more"), which is very similar to the way he describes his father's response to him as a child. Importantly, Mr. V links this pattern to a disruption in his mood ("I feel really bad, like nervous") and a degradation of his relationship with his employer.

Although recognizing that there will likely be unavoidable enactments in which Mr. V experiences her via the lens of this transference, Dr. D notes that this treatment will be one in which reasonable goals should be set and the patient's efforts not only encouraged but also acknowledged.

Inquire Specifically About the Patient's Experiences With Psychiatric Caregiving

Based on what she has heard, it is not clear whether Mr. V's mood lability is characterological or bipolar, although Dr. D has a sense that there is at least some characterological contribution. However, biomedical diagnosis is not the priority of this first meeting because there does not appear to be an urgent need to adjust the treatment. Rather, the prescriber considers that the primary task of this meeting is establishing the alliance and a way of working. At this point, she chooses to make a more or less explicit link between parental and pharmacological caregiving and inquires about the patient's experience with psychiatric caregiving.

> Dr. D: It sounds like your basic experiences with authority figures have been really complicated. This makes me wonder how your relationships with doctors have been. I wonder about the particular things that worked or didn't work with the doctors who saw you before me.
>
> Mr. V: There have only been a couple. I can't stand it when a doctor is really arrogant, when they think they always know better. I mean, I think Dr. N was okay. He was my last doctor. He tried to help me get off some of my medications. I think he knew what he was doing, but half the time he couldn't remember my medications, and he kept forgetting about my pain. He would tell me to exercise and stuff. That would bug me because I can't.
>
> Dr. D: But it sounds like you thought he was okay. Or did I misunderstand?
>
> Mr. V: No. He was pretty busy, so I kind of understand. At least he respected me and listened to me. When I called him, he called me back, and he was trying to help me get off my medications.
>
> Dr. D: It sounds like there were some others.
>
> Mr. V: My doctor before that, Dr. M, was awful! I saw him after the hospital. He had me on, like, three antipsychotics.
>
> Dr. D: Three antipsychotics?
>
> Mr. V: He was all "medications are the answer" and always saying why the next medicine was going to be the right one. He was so full of himself, but the only thing he ever really did was make me fat.
>
> Dr. D: You didn't like the way he was prescribing for you. Did you ever tell him this?
>
> Mr. V: [Sarcastically] Well, *he* was the doctor. And besides, I think I wanted to have hope. He showed me how he was going to fix the different brain chemicals, and he was so sure. I wanted to believe him, but I still always kind of thought he was full of it. Eventually, I just kind of gave up, and I stopped going and stopped taking them because it didn't seem like they were helping.

Again, inquiring about the patient's feelings regarding previous providers has taken less than 3 minutes, but it has given the prescriber a wealth of information about how to approach this patient and the prescribing task in a way that is most likely to support a working alliance. Mr. V provided further evidence that negative paternal transferences may easily interfere with the working alliance and that he will be attuned to anything that seems arrogant or as though the prescriber knows better. He has also suggested that he is attuned to maternal transferences of being preoccupied, but like with his mother, he is more prepared to forgive such lapses of attention. Perhaps most important, he has revealed that when there are problems with his prescriber, he tries to suppress or ignore them but remains covertly frustrated.

A psychologically astute prescriber will recognize that much of this patient's orientation toward caregivers and authority figures is not fully conscious. In addition to exploring Mr. V's conscious attitudes, Dr. D will also listen for his unconscious or implicit authority relations. Does he appear to operate as a partner and equal, engaging concerns and making his wishes known, or does he acquiesce, passively resist, or surreptitiously attempt to control treatment by controlling the information available to the prescriber? Listening to both the words and the music, Dr. D will not only gather this information from the history but also assess how these dynamics are operating in the here and now.

Inquire Specifically About the Patient's Feelings About Taking Medications

Dr. D decides to explore Mr. V's feelings about medications, ideally before the end of this hour. When Mr. V mentions how much he valued Dr. N's approach, which included a focus on deprescribing, this is the perfect opportunity to inquire further about his feelings regarding taking medications.

Dr. D: It sounds like one of the things that worked with Dr. N was that he was trying to help you get off of medications. That makes me wonder how much getting off of medications is a goal you have with me, as well.

Mr. V: I don't know. I think my feelings have changed a little. I just want to do what helps me. I want to get on with my life. I'm tired of my mood swings.

Dr. D: But you wanted to get off of medications, at least in the past.

Mr. V: I wasn't sure that they were helping.

Dr. D: I wonder what it's like for you to take medications.

Mr. V: Well, I really hate feeling dependent. That's what I hate the most. I'd really like to not be on any medications, but I understand if I might need some.

Dr. D: I think this is really important, and I agree with you. I'd also like to find ways to have you on the least amount of medications possible. I think if you can find ways to do for yourself what the medications do, then that's the best option. I don't know enough yet about your troubles to know how to do that, but I think it's something we can work toward.

Mr. V: I'd like that. Maybe we can start with the Latuda, or anything. I don't really know what anything is doing.

Dr. D: Hopefully, we can find out a little more about how you really are struggling, and then we can make decisions based on that.

Mr. V: Uh huh.

Dr. D: You said that depending on medications was what you hated the most. Does that mean there are other things that you hate?

Mr. V: Well, I hate that they make me fat. I'm not really like this. My normal weight is about 150. Sometimes, when I first start them, they make me feel better, but then, when I gain weight, that has the opposite effect, and it makes me more depressed.

This inquiry into Mr. V's feelings about medications has exposed some of the more salient sources of his ambivalence about medications that may interfere with medication adherence or promote nocebogenesis. First and foremost, the patient is concerned about dependency. He also believes medications have harmed him, mostly by contributing to weight gain. Furthermore, although he was more opposed to medications previously, he is still not convinced they have been helpful, despite seeming to decompensate after discontinuing them unilaterally.

Explore Secondary Gains That May Contribute to Treatment Resistance

The assessment of potential sources of ambivalence has so far focused on the patient's ambivalence about medications and treaters. Dr. D is also interested to know if Mr. V is ambivalent about illness itself.

Dr. D: I wonder if you have thoughts about whether there's anything you might lose if treatment worked.

Mr. V: My self-respect.

Dr. D: Your self-respect?

Mr. V: Yeah, then I wouldn't be able to feel that I did it myself.

In this case, although the patient indicates his ambivalence about being helped by medications, he does not give an indication of being attached to his illness or being aware of deriving secondary gains. What should Dr. D do about her patient's ambivalence? Mr. V has already established that it is not helpful to take one side of the ambivalence, for instance, talking the medications up as his previous prescriber had done. Rather, she elects to join Mr. V's reasonable goal of only taking as much medication as is necessary. In doing so, the prescriber is working to foster a positive working alliance in which she takes the patient's treatment goal(s) seriously, with an ear to "how is the patient right."

Negotiate a Working Alliance

There is still some negotiation to be done in this case in establishing a way of working together that includes the basic principles of psychodynamic psychopharmacology and acknowledges the importance of meaning, relationships, and patient authority in this treatment. Although this does not have to be done in the first hour, it is useful, when possible, to do this before beginning active treatment, even if that active treatment does not involve active medication changes. Establishing a shared understanding of the impact of psychosocial factors on pharmacotherapy outcomes authorizes prescribers to notice aspects of patients' psychology that might adversely affect outcomes. Without such authorization, patients may more easily feel intruded upon or even blamed.

> Dr. D: We only have a few minutes left, and I think this is a good time to segue into talking a bit more about how I work and how I hope we can work together. First of all, you may have already noticed that I'm interested in the bigger picture, not just your symptoms. In fact, in this way of working, my goal is not necessarily to eradicate your symptoms. We are working at trying to get you to where you want to get in your life, using medications or maybe even taking them away. For example, say it took 400 mg of Seroquel to completely eradicate your anxiety. Now you would be without anxiety, but you might well be too sedated for work or school. We would try to make adjustments that fit your life. Does that sound okay?
>
> Mr. V: Yes.

Provide Psychoeducation About the Psychosocial Dimension of Psychopharmacology

In the engagement phase, psychoeducation (Table 16–5) is one of the tools for empowering patients and supporting the alliance. Going beyond education about conditions and their treatments, prescribers should also talk to patients about basic concepts involving psychosocial aspects of pharmacotherapy. This helps provide a rationale for this way of working, ensures that patients are informed participants, highlights the role that patients play in optimizing outcomes, and can be used to highlight psychosocial factors that may undercut the effort of pharmacotherapy. For example, for patients who are prone to side effects, education might cover the role of powerlessness and negative expectations in nocebo responsiveness.

> Dr. D: Another thing that may be different from what you're used to is that I'm going to be paying attention to what things mean to you in treatment because evidence suggests that much of what happens with medications has to do with other things, like the placebo effect. You've heard of the placebo effect, right?
>
> Mr. V: Yeah. Sure.
>
> Dr. D: There's evidence to suggest that the placebo effect may contribute more than half of the effect of some medications. And "placebo" does

Table 16–5. Psychoeducation emphasizing patients' role in effective pharmacotherapy

Placebo effects

Nocebo effects

Role of patient preferences

Readiness to change

Benefits of a strong alliance

not mean unreal or imaginary. Placebo effects are real. They can cure ulcers, lower blood pressure, and decrease pain transmission in nerve fibers. Sometimes this kind of effect is what makes the difference between when treatments work and when they don't. That's why we'll also be paying attention to what treatment means for you.

Mr. V: [Nodding] That's interesting.

Specifically Authorize the Patient to Address Problems in the Alliance

Given the importance of the alliance as a therapeutic tool and the struggles patients may have with straightforwardly assuming authority for their treatment, it is helpful to emphasize the benefits of a good working alliance.

Dr. D: We also know that a treatment that you want works better than one that you don't, and there are a lot of other ways that meaning affects medications. This one is especially important: evidence suggests that medications from a doctor you work well with work better than medications from a doctor you don't, so the better we work together, the more benefit I think you can get from your medications. This means that it's very important for you to tell me when I'm doing something that doesn't work for you. Actually, I count on it. I need that from you if I'm going to do my job effectively. Do you think you can do that?

Mr. V: Yeah, I think so. I don't think that any doctor has ever said that to me before.

Dr. D: That's good to know. I know it's not always that easy. You've already told me that you can kind of bite your tongue when you don't like what authority figures are doing, but I really mean it that I count on you to tell me when I'm getting it wrong.

Mr. V: Okay. I really will try.

At this point, prescriber and patient have reached a tentative agreement of working that will seriously consider both the biomedical and psychosocial aspects of pharmacotherapy. This will, of course, be a work in progress, with such negotiations occurring in an ongoing way as either participant departs from or wishes to depart from the agreed-upon way of working. By encouraging Mr. V to protest, if he needs to, Dr. D explicitly authorizes him to request changes in the terms of the agreement and to notice when she has, for her own reasons, departed from providing such care. Given that part of the agreement is focused on the patient's growth and developmental goals, it also authorizes the prescriber to explore countertherapeutic uses of treatment, such as those that might lead to chronicity (as discussed in Chapter 6).

> Dr. D: Our time is just about up. Unless we have to, I'd rather not make any medication changes today. There's a lot going on right now, with you coming into treatment. If you felt better next week, or worse, I think it would be very hard for us to know if it was because of the medicine or because of other things.
>
> Mr. V: No. That's good.
>
> Dr. D: One of the things that I hope will happen in this treatment is that you will have a clearer sense of what medications do and don't do. Normally, that's why I try to change only one medication at a time. If we change more than one thing at a time, it's really hard to know what's doing what. One of the ways you get to be more in charge of your treatment is by understanding what really works. Is that okay?
>
> Mr. V: Yeah.
>
> Dr. D: Okay. One last thing. I just wanted to ask how you think this meeting went. How it felt meeting with me. Was there anything I did that didn't feel like it worked for you?
>
> Mr. V: No, no. I think this was good. I liked it. It makes sense.
>
> Dr. D: Great, but please let me know if or when that changes. One thing that would help me is if you can bring a list of past medication trials next time so we can think about what worked and what didn't. I'd like to see you in a week so we can complete the initial evaluation. Would that work for you?

Dr. D recognizes that ongoing work is needed to develop a deeper understanding of how intrapsychic and interpersonal dynamics impact the patient's capacity for optimal use of medications. At this time, however, she thinks she has accomplished many of the goals of the engagement phase of psychodynamic psychopharmacology. By avoiding a mind-body split and promoting a patient-centered focus, she has engaged the patient in a way that focuses on how his symptoms interfere with his functioning and achievement of developmental goals. In understanding *who* her patient is (as opposed to *what* her patient is), the prescriber has gotten some understanding of his broader goals and has developed a sense of some of the transference-based, interpersonal patterns that may manifest in their therapeutic relationship, potentially fueling Mr. V's ambivalence about and resistance to treatment. She has made a basic assessment of his ambivalence about medications, although she still has questions regarding the ways in which he may be ambivalent about his symptoms. There are hints that Mr. V may use his symptoms to escape the burden of perfectionism when he thinks he is not performing adequately, insofar as having a medical problem may absolve him of some guilt or shame. This is something Dr. D hopes to explore further in the next appointment and beyond in an effort to understand if Mr. V uses treatment in unconscious, countertherapeutic ways.

Furthermore, in this session, Dr. D has done several things to establish a solid working alliance. By focusing on the patient's life history and larger developmental goals, she has demonstrated an interest in him as a person. She has tried to convey, nonverbally, some warmth, openness, empathy, and investment in his goals. She has also limited her use of mediating technology by taking brief notes with pen and paper. Furthermore, Dr. D has begun to explicitly join places where their interests align, beyond the idea of symptom relief, for example, noting a shared interest in using only as much medication as necessary to achieve Mr. V's goals. Finally, she has offered the patient a framework for understanding how psychological and interpersonal factors impact pharmacotherapy and suggested that he take an active role in his recovery, in part, by helping attend to the pharmacotherapeutic alliance.

In their next session, they will focus more on diagnostic issues and pharmacotherapy as Dr. D works toward forming an overall diagnosis that integrates her understanding of Mr. V as both subject and object. By the end of that session, she anticipates achieving enough clarity about the patient's diagnosis and treatment to allow her to make preliminary medical recommendations. Furthermore, she believes she will understand enough about Mr. V's ways of relating to treatment that she will have a sense of *what* to prescribe and *how* to prescribe it.

Follow-Up Intake Session

In their second meeting, Dr. D first wants to know how things are going and whether there have been any significant changes since they last met. Here, she is trying to determine whether there is any reason to shift the focus from a comprehensive biopsychosocial assessment to attend to any urgent psychiatric concerns.

> Dr. D: Today we were going to think a little more about how to understand and treat the issues you're up against. Before we get to that, I wanted to ask, how are things going? Is there anything that you're dealing with right now?
> Mr. V: I think things are going okay. I mean, I haven't had any big problems.
> Dr. D: You're getting settled.
> Mr. V: Uh-huh. I'm trying to not hide behind my mask, working on trying to not be fake.

Dr. D: That's interesting. I'm not sure that I know what you mean. I didn't quite appreciate that you wear a mask.

Mr. V: Well, like you said last week, I try so hard to do good, but I try to keep the bad things to myself. I don't usually let people know so much when there is a problem.

Dr. D notices that this is an interesting way for Mr. V to start the second appointment, and she registers that what she said to him in the previous appointment was, in some way, emotionally important for him. Although she could delve deeper into the topic of mask wearing, Dr. D believes she has already made a basic assessment of the ways Mr. V has difficulty allowing others to see his struggles until he is at the point of collapse, and she has stressed the importance of addressing problems with pharmacotherapy early. She thinks that exploring this further would detract from the current pharmacotherapeutic task and might also confuse the boundary between psychotherapy and pharmacotherapy.

On the other hand, there might be more to be gained, from a pharmacotherapy perspective, in exploring the doctor–patient relationship further. Mindful of the transference paradigm that Mr. V described relating to a demanding and harsh paternal figure, Dr. D wonders whether Mr. V believes he must acquiesce to a judging father figure or if his proclamation about being more honest expresses a positive and trusting attitude about the invitation to express his concerns. All of this passes through her mind in a matter of seconds, and she might not have even noticed these thoughts except that she has been working at staying attuned to the meaning of the pharmacotherapy interaction. Ultimately, she thinks the ways that her patient experiences her (as bad or good) will become clearer over time and be addressed in the course of the ongoing treatment, especially to the extent his feelings present as a resistance to the optimal use of psychiatric treatment. However, before shifting gears toward a focus on greater diagnostic clarity, Dr. D also knows that Mr. V needs his healthy strivings to be acknowledged. She believes that explicitly acknowledging his efforts will foster the pharmacotherapeutic alliance, not only by avoiding a known pitfall of the negative transference (feeling easily angered that his efforts are unappreciated or appropriated) and promoting a good feeling about the relationship but also by reinforcing the patient's agency.

Dr. D: Well, that does sound like an important bit of work you're doing with yourself…and it may be challenging, too, to try to do things in a different way. I hope we can pay attention to this and that this will be a place where you can let me know when you're struggling, especially if that struggle relates to something with me, because it may help your medications work better.

Mr. V: Yeah. Me, too. I think it will be.

Dr. D: Is there anything else that seems important since our meeting last Monday?

Mr. V: No, not really.

Dr. D: Well then, I wanted to start with something you said last Monday. I noticed you mentioned bipolar disorder but you mostly talked about depression. It makes me wonder, what do you think about being diagnosed as bipolar? Is it your general sense that this diagnosis fits?

Dr. D is beginning to move toward gaining diagnostic clarity, but by asking for Mr. V's own diagnostic assessment, she is also trying to gain a better understanding of his relationship with diagnosis. She knows that if they can agree on the diagnosis, her patient is about twice as likely to adhere to the recommended regimen (Woolley et al. 2010).

Mr. V: That's a good question. Sometimes I don't know. When I was first diagnosed, I didn't agree with it. For sure. I didn't like the idea and didn't want to have to take any medications. But then, it's true that my mood goes up and down all the time. I can never know what it's going to be like, so I guess it fits.

Dr. D: Could you say a bit more about how your moods go up and down? There are lots of ways that this can happen, Maybe we can start with how this diagnosis first came about.

As Dr. D drills down on the specifics, she learns that the diagnosis was first broached when Mr. V was in college, as a result of disciplinary action following a drunken fight on campus. He had been referred to the college counseling service for assessment and was started on Seroquel but did not take it for more than a few days. When she inquires why he did not follow through with treatment, Mr. V notes that he disagreed with the diagnosis and believed the medication was punitive. He also hated the idea of taking medications, especially because he always thought his father wanted him to take medications as a child. Mr. V adds that he was hospitalized with a possible manic episode following another drunken altercation that year. Specifically, he threw a chair through a glass door at the student union and then tried to steal a campus police car. Although he has no memory of the event, he was told that he had been hospitalized by campus police after making suicidal statements.

Dr. D observes that Mr. V had not mentioned this second hospitalization, and Mr. V clarifies that he was never admitted; he had spent the night in the emergency room but had been released the following day. As in any diagnostically focused evaluation, Dr. D tries to understand whether these episodes of dyscontrol always involved alcohol, and she inquires as to whether Mr. V has experienced symptoms of bipolarity since he became sober. In response to her focused questioning, Mr. V reports that there are periods, usually lasting 1–4 days, when he feels a lift in mood, an increased sense of hopefulness, and an increase in future-oriented, goal-directed behavior (e.g., making plans to study differently). He believes such periods of increased mood and energy happen several times a year. He also reports increased impulsiveness during such episodes. For example, he admits occasionally gambling during these periods, which is uncharacteristic. In response to further inquiry, Mr. V clarifies that his gambling, although atypical, is not out of control, and he has never lost more than $200–$300. Except for some things that happened when he was drinking, he has never encountered negative consequences while in these states. He reports that he can be irritable but does not think it is radically different from when he gets aggravated at other times. He also believes these states allow him to be more social but has never received feedback about being more talkative. He also does not believe his sleep is more disrupted in these states.

On inquiry, Mr. V suggests that he has been less reactive when he takes mood-stabilizing medications. In fact, he has been prescribed quite a few, including quetiapine, risperidone, olanzapine, lithium, valproate, aripiprazole, and, currently, lurasidone and lamotrigine. He interrupted many of these medication trials because he took issue with his diagnosis and felt stigmatized by being on medications or by side effects (e.g., tremor from lithium). He also stopped medications on several occasions because he felt sedated and was upset about weight gain. Medication discontinuation was generally done without consulting his doctor, although it had been better with his most recent prescriber. In addition, Mr. V underwent several trials of low-dosage antidepressants. Although he experienced fewer side effects, he prematurely (and often unilaterally) stopped these trials as well. Furthermore, exploration reveals that Mr. V almost always believed he did not need the medication, especially when he began feeling better. He adamantly proclaims that he did not want to be reliant on medication to feel better, although he also recognizes the impossible bind this conflict engenders.

To recap, the primary task of this portion of the evaluation is to seek diagnostic clarity. In many respects, this task is no different from a more biomedically focused assessment. What may be different is that the prescriber also asks about the phenomenology of the experience and what meaning the patient makes of these symptoms. She ascertains that Mr. V does not experience these brief periods of increased activity as out of the blue or out of control; rather, when he feels transiently more hopeful and energized, he feels pressed to do as much as he can in the anticipation that this feeling is unlikely to last.

For further diagnostic clarification, Dr. D inquires about any family history of psychiatric illness. Apart from his brother, who has autism spectrum disorder, Mr. V has a cousin on his maternal side who was also diagnosed with bipolar disorder, depression and anxiety are scattered throughout the maternal lineage, and a paternal uncle died of complications of alcoholism. While exploring the family history, Dr. D asks about his family's attitudes toward mental illness and treatment because ideas and concerns that are deeply embedded in a family context may shape his experience of illness or create family resistances to treatment that Mr. V will have to face.

Mr. V: That's the thing that doesn't make sense. On my dad's side, I don't really know what's going on because they don't talk about that kind of thing. It's like hush-hush. They never talk about my uncle or my grandfather.

Dr. D: Your grandfather?

Mr. V: Yeah, I forgot to say, my grandfather died in a car accident. I don't know what happened, but my aunt told one of my cousins that she thought it might have been suicide.

Dr. D: What do you think?

Mr. V: Like I said [with a hint of irritation], I don't know. My dad never talked about anything like that, but it could be.

Dr. D: You just surprised me a bit with your grandfather, but you were trying to say that there was something that didn't make sense about how your family thinks about psychiatric troubles.

Mr. V: Yeah. With my dad and his family, it's all hush-hush, but with me, it's like he really wants me to take medications, and it's like he wants to tell people that his son has bipolar.

Dr. D: And it seems like you might have some feelings about that.

Mr. V: Yeah. It's nobody's business but my own, but it's like he kind of gets off on it. Maybe because he thinks it's my mom's fault. When I first got diagnosed, he always used to say that it was because of my mom's "weak genes."

Dr. D: What do you think about that?

Mr. V: I think my dad's an asshole!

This exchange has failed to fully clarify Mr. V's diagnosis. A number of things in the history suggest bipolar disorder, but atypical elements, such as the brief duration of episodes and, especially, the absence of sleep disruption argue against it. The family history is also unclear in this regard. A paternal cousin has been diagnosed with bipolar disorder, but it is unknown on what grounds. There may be more psychopathology in the paternal lineage, but this has never been discussed. Nonetheless, this exchange has further illuminated some of the family dynamics that may complicate Mr. V's relation to treatment. One example is the sense of shame that has been quietly passed on to him through the family's secretiveness. More overtly, shame is also projected onto Mr. V through his father's contemptuous equation of bipolar disorder with "weak" maternal genes. Mr. V has also raised the question of whether manic defenses are in operation rather than true bipolarity. Dr. D hopes that Mr. V's history of medication response will offer further clues as to the most accurate diagnosis.

Dr. D: I want to return to something you said last week. You mentioned that, when your doctor, the one you didn't like...

Mr. V: Dr. M.

Dr. D: Right. You mentioned that you just stopped taking your medications. Do you remember how that went and why you decided to go back on them?

Mr. V: Yeah. I didn't really notice anything after I stopped. I lost a bunch of weight, but it didn't really make a difference in my mood or anything.

Dr. D: But you went back on medications...

Mr. V: Yeah, I think that was, like, the year before I graduated. I had another episode. I got into a big argument with my dad.

Dr. D: What happened?

Mr. V: I got really mad and threw a plate toward him. It wasn't at him. I wasn't trying to hit him, but he ran to the phone to call the police. I freaked out and tried to grab the phone, and he hit me with it. I ended up getting three stitches in my head, but I pushed him into a wall. I scared the hell out of my mom, too. I lost it. The police came, and I ended up in the ER again and got interviewed by psych. They agreed not to admit me if I went back on my meds. That's when I decided just to take my meds.

Dr. D: Were there other things going on? Was alcohol involved this time, too? Or other stressors?

Mr. V: No, this was after the car thing at school, so I was sober.

Dr. D: And since you started taking your medications again, have there been other problems like this? You mentioned being hospitalized.

Mr. V: Well, that's what I meant. I went to the hospital to get evaluated, but they didn't admit me.

Dr. D inquires further about subsequent mood lability. Mr. V intermittently experiences brief periods of increased mood and impulsivity, but nothing that has resulted in adverse consequences. He also reports periods of irritability, but this seems to be closely associated with periods of increased stress, feeling overwhelmed, or fears of judgment. His irritability tends to manifest when he is feeling more depressed, and it is this that has primarily interfered with Mr. V's functioning in age-appropriate roles.

From the history gathered thus far, it remains unclear as to whether this patient has a bipolar diathesis. If there is one, he does not have a history of full mania; much of the mood lability seems explainable by the recognition that he has some narcissistic vulnerabilities and difficulties with affect management that are characteristic of a Cluster B characterological disorder.

Negotiate a Shared Understanding

To ground the treatment in a strong pharmacotherapeutic alliance, Dr. D shares her current understanding with Mr. V. Negotiating a shared understanding is pivotal because it more than doubles the likelihood that patients will adhere to the negotiated regimen (Woolley et al. 2010). In keeping with basic tenets of psychodynamic psychopharmacology (Table 16–6), Dr. D tries to do this in a way that 1) recognizes the true complexity of the interrelation of biological and psychosocial factors contributing to illness expression, 2) attends to potential meanings of symptoms, and 3) emphasizes that the patient's attitudes and behaviors can shape treatment outcome.

> Dr. D: So, Mr. V, let me tell you what I understand from what you're telling me because I'd like to make sure we're on the same page about how we understand this. I think it's clear that you've had depressive episodes, and it's your depression that seems to be the biggest problem, at least recently.
>
> Mr. V: Totally. The depression is the worst part.
>
> Dr. D: But I think it's much more complicated than this. If you have bipolar disorder—and I'm not completely sure that you fully meet criteria for that diagnosis—I think it's fairly mild. You have some mood swings that sound like bipolar disorder, but you said your sleep isn't usually disrupted when you're in an up mood.
>
> Mr. V: Yeah. I don't know. Maybe sometimes…but no, probably not that much. It's always kind of bad, anyway.
>
> Dr. D: So, this is something we'll keep an eye on. I think it will become clearer over time because if there really aren't worse problems with sleep when your mood is up, then it's probably not bipolar disorder. But I also want to notice that there are some other things that might make it more confusing. First of all, you said that when you're feeling better, you want to take advantage of that and try to do as much as you can while it lasts. That could be a sign of bipolar disorder, but it could also be something that *you* do…kind of speeding yourself up to try to outrun bad feelings. Do you know what I mean?
>
> Mr. V: Yeah. I don't know if I said this, but, when I'm feeling good, it's like I want to do as much as I can because I don't know when I'm going to feel depressed again, and it will be harder to do. I don't know if that's exactly the same thing.
>
> Dr. D: That's the kind of thing I'm talking about. There are also the ways that your mood goes up and down. It's faster than usual in bipolar disorder, and the way I hear it, it's often in response to things happening around you, you know? Like, when you're stressed or not meeting the high standards you have, the bottom can kind of drop out.
>
> Mr. V: Uh huh, yeah.
>
> Dr. D: And it seems your mood may also bump up when good things happen that make you feel better about yourself. I think this says that your ups and downs are complicated and affected by things like how you handle emotions, especially bad ones, and how issues around self-esteem can really affect how you feel and how you function.

Develop a Medication Plan

With the understanding that "the doctor is the drug" (Balint 1957), the whole engagement up to this point has been treatment. However, having come to some kind of shared understanding (as imprecise as it is), the prescriber and

Table 16–6. Negotiating a working alliance

Develop patient-centered goals.	Focus on life-historical context of the psychiatric complaint, demonstrating interest in the patient as a person.
	Elicit and engage patient's understanding of his or her struggles.
	Incorporate patient's developmental goals in the treatment goals, focusing not only on mental illness but also on mental health.
Negotiate a biopsychosocial frame that emphasizes the role of psychological factors in treatment outcome.	Actively explore psychosocial factors that might impact medication response in order to demonstrate their importance.
	Show realistic humility about the potency of medication.
	Provide psychoeducation about the interaction of meaning and medication.
	Find meaning, whenever possible, in symptoms or treatment resistance.
	Provide a therapeutic rationale for leveraging the psychosocial dimensions of pharmacotherapy.
Emphasize the role of patient agency.	While addressing unrealistic hopes for pharmacotherapy, emphasize hopefulness of mobilizing patient agency.
	Elicit treatment preferences.
	Offer choices that permit expression of preferences (and explore the meaning of those choices).
	Actively question patient's deauthorizing assumptions.
Tend the prescriber–patient bond.	Demonstrate respect, warmth, and interest in the patient and other evidence-based behaviors that promote alliance.
	Maintain a nonauthoritarian stance.
	Emphasize the importance of the alliance for supporting outcomes.
	Specifically authorize patient to engage prescriber about prescriber behaviors that weaken the alliance.
Identify and address potential resistances to treatment.	Explore patient's history of interactions with caregiving and authority figures.
	Explore patient's feelings about medications, paying attention to negative or ambivalent feelings.
	Explore what the patient might lose if treatment is effective.
	Name repeating patterns that have the potential to undercut treatment.

the patient must now begin making mutually acceptable plans for treatment. In the routine practice of psychodynamic psychopharmacology, the medication plan involves not only selecting an appropriate medication regimen based on sound evidence but also incorporating psychosocial factors to optimize outcomes. Attention to psychosocial factors can empower patients in many ways, such as collaboratively anticipating the dynamics that disrupted prior treatment. Careful negotiation of a treatment plan typically involves 1) maintaining realistic humility regarding the likely benefits of medication; 2) emphasizing the psychosocial factors within patients' control that could optimize outcomes; 3) involving patients in medical decision making and responding, when reasonable, to the patients' preferences; and 4) specifying paths of action if anticipated dynamics emerge that have the potential to interfere with treatment.

Maintain Realistic Humility About the Potency of Medications

In this case, it is easy to maintain realistic humility about the effects of medications. At best, Mr. V has only experienced a partial response to multiple medication trials, so he likely will not prefer an overly optimistic approach (Priebe et al. 2017), as is typically the case with the treatment-resistant patients for whom psychodynamic psychopharmacology is specifically adapted.

Emphasize the Patient's Role in Promoting Good Outcomes

Furthermore, given the formulation that there is a characterological contribution to Mr. V's affective instability, it will be important for Dr. D to emphasize ways in which the patient can contribute to a positive outcome above and beyond the pharmacological effects of medication. Often, this includes efforts such as maintaining a healthy lifestyle and social rhythms to improve mood and promote stability, as well as staying aware of sources of ambivalence about treatment and bringing those into the prescriber–patient relationship. When patients have significant ambivalence regarding their health or caregiving (as in this case), use treatment countertherapeutically, or have contributing deficits in affect competence, adjunctive psychotherapy is also recommended.

> Dr. D: Like I said, I think your diagnosis is complicated. If there is bipolar disorder, it's probably mild. But you do have other problems that have to do with how you manage bad feelings. I think the way your father was so hard on you, you know, had a major effect that you're still dealing with. Your self-esteem took a beating. Then, on top of that, you ended

up feeling that you had to compensate by being perfect. I think those things affect your mood a lot. It's hard to ever really feel good when you have such perfectionistic demands. And when things hurt your self-esteem, I think that probably sends your mood careening, so there are a lot of ups and downs just from that. Medications can help with this, too, and it's basically a lot of the same medications we might use for mild bipolar disorder. That's some of the good news. The even better news is that we can get more benefit from your medications when we pay attention to the psychological part of things. It may even turn out that, in the end, you could learn to manage on very little medication if you learn how to deal with bad feelings. I think that, in your case, it will be helpful to get back into therapy to work on perfectionism and self-esteem issues, because that will probably help your mood as much as medications.

Involve the Patient in Medical Decision Making

With regard to a medication plan, the question is whether to begin lowering medications, as per Mr. V's expressed interest, or to hold still while establishing a baseline that will help make things clearer in the future. Although Mr. V expresses a preference to be off medications, there is also a third option, in Dr. D's opinion, which is to add a low-dosage antidepressant in the context of residual depressive symptoms. This is not a decision for the prescriber to make on her own. Instead, she lays out the reasonable options, including the significant risks and benefits of each approach, and gives the patient an opportunity to shape medical decision making.

Mr. V: So, what do you think I should do? Which is best?

Dr. D: Well, that is a complicated question. All three options are reasonable. Like I said before, if there's one that you prefer, it might work best.

Mr. V: Well, I don't think I want to start something new. Not right now. I'd rather try to get off of things. I'd kind of like to make a new start, you know?

Dr. D: Okay, but I do wonder if your wanting to stop medications may be part of the problem, too. I thought maybe that antidepressants helped, but if you listen to what you told me, you stopped them as soon as you started feeling better, so you never really gave them a chance to work fully.

Mr. V: So, should I start an antidepressant?

Dr. D: No. I'm not disagreeing with your plan. I'm just keeping things complicated. I think it makes sense to see how you can manage with lower medications. If we do it together, and go slow, that will give us a clearer sense of how much the medications are helping. Especially if therapy helps, we may be able to get away with less medication. If feeling down ends up getting in your way, there is always time to explore other options. I just want you to get a good start here.

Dr. D suggests discontinuing the clonazepam because Mr. V takes it so infrequently, and she believes there are better options for treating anxiety that have fewer liabilities and less chance of dependency, which is a concern for Mr. V. He readily agrees to this but is also interested in discontinuing his lurasidone, which is at a marginally subtherapeutic level. They make a plan to halve the dosage, and as long as that goes well, to discuss discontinuing in a month. Mr. V is pleased with this plan.

Inoculate the Patient Against Dynamics That Undercut Growth

If there are anticipated complications based on the patient's history or dynamics, these should also be included in the informal treatment agreement. Examples might include unilateral treatment discontinuation, avoidance of conflict, or overreliance on sedating medications to manage negative affects. In Mr. V's case, several key factors have been identified. He has a history of medication nonadherence. This appears to be related both to side effects (sedation, weight gain) and to concerns about weakness and dependency. His unilateral decisions are often unconstrained by a sense of mutual trust. Expecting unpleasant interactions in the face of potential conflict, he deals with this by withdrawing and does not voice any complaints or concerns when they emerge. Dr. D tries to negotiate an agreement for how they might attend to such treatment-interfering dynamics.

> Dr. D: Based on your history, you may be in a hurry to discontinue your medications. I think you can end up pushing yourself like your dad pushed you, and that didn't always turn out so well. Because we're trying to get a clear idea about what works and what doesn't and avoid other problems, like rebound symptoms, I hope that if you want to make changes to the plan, you'll hold off until we can discuss it. Does that make sense?
>
> Mr. V: For sure. I can stick to the plan as long as I know that we're headed in the right direction.
>
> Dr. D: Last week we talked about how important it is to let me know if there are things that aren't working or if it feels like you don't agree with something or even if I have said something that you don't like. I really mean it that I need to hear those things.
>
> Mr. V: No. I got it. I think that's good. I can do that.

Develop a Psychodynamic Formulation

At the conclusion of this session, Dr. D offers to facilitate a connection with a therapist that she trusts, which Mr. V accepts, and they make a plan to meet in 1 month to explore further reductions in lurasidone. In her note, she includes a provisional psychodynamic formulation of factors relevant to Mr. V's use of pharmacotherapy:

> Growing up in a demeaning and demanding environment in which his parents were not emotional resources, and feeling that he needed to compensate for his autistic brother, Mr. V was left feeling unseen and inadequate. As an adult, he repeats this pattern through unattainable personal standards and ruthless self-criticism. He expects others to respond to him in kind, leading him to mask his vulnerability or to lash out in ways that are significantly disruptive. Having little expectation that caregivers will listen to and support him, he adopts a counterdependent stance and may be tempted to take medication decisions into his own hands. In this way, medications may get recruited as symbols of personal weakness or as weapons to communicate bad feelings. At the same time, he may grasp at biologized explanations defensively to avoid feelings of shame.

Key Points

- The nature of the alliance developed in the first few sessions may determine how easy it will be to confront meaning-based problems in pharmacotherapy at later stages, when treatment resistance emerges.

- A focused developmental history that includes early models of caregiving and characteristic relationship patterns may help prescribers predict and address likely interferences with the healthy use of medications.

- Inquiring about the patient's experiences with and feelings about taking medications may also help prescribers predict and address likely interferences.

- Patients' active participation as partners may be enhanced by psychoeducation about the psychosocial determinants of pharmacotherapy outcome.

- A negotiated treatment plan should emphasize patients' role in their own recovery.

References

Balint M: The Doctor and His Patient and the Illness. London, Pitman, 1957

Freud S: On beginning the treatment (further recommendations on the technique of psycho-analysis I) (1913), in Standard Edition of the Complete Psychological Works of Sigmund Freud, Vol 12. Translated and edited by Strachey J. London, Hogarth, 1958, pp 121–144

Priebe S, Ramjaun G, Strappelli N, et al: Do patients prefer optimistic or cautious psychiatrists? An experimental study with new and long-term patients. BMC Psychiatry 17(1):26, 2017 28095888

Woolley SB, Fredman L, Goethe JW, et al: Hospital patients' perceptions during treatment and early discontinuation of serotonin selective reuptake inhibitor antidepressants. J Clin Psychopharmacol 30(6):716–719, 2010 21105288

Zuroff DC, Blatt SJ, Sotsky SM, et al: Relation of therapeutic alliance and perfectionism to outcome in brief outpatient treatment of depression. J Consult Clin Psychol 68(1):114–124, 2000 10710846

• CHAPTER 17 •

The Maintenance Phase

Ultimately, and precisely in the deepest and most important matters,
we are unspeakably alone; and many things must happen, many things
must go right, a whole constellation of events must be fulfilled, for one
human being to successfully advise or help another.

—Rainer Maria Rilke, *Letters to a Young Poet*

In the engagement phase, an alliance is negotiated that acknowledges that psychological and interpersonal factors play an important role in psychiatric illness and response to medications. The tasks of this phase tend to follow an established path, as Freud noted in his chess metaphor (Freud 1913/1958; quoted in Chapter 16). The potency of patients' efforts, both conscious and unconscious, is recognized, empowering them to be agents in their own recovery. When developing an overall diagnosis, prescribers also begin to identify personal and interpersonal dynamics that might contribute to treatment resistance. This initial agreement is the backdrop against which the work of the maintenance phase proceeds.

The maintenance phase is governed more by principles and is adapted more specifically to patients' unique needs and dynamics. Within this patient-centered and psychodynamically informed framework, medication choices and how medications and diagnoses are discussed are shaped by patients' developmental goals. Psychodynamic psychopharmacologists remain mindful of opportunities to emphasize the patients' role in optimizing pharmacotherapy outcomes and strive to develop an alliance in which patients' desires harness their own pharmacological expertise. This is more complicated than it sounds because, from a psychodynamic perspective, patients have multiple and conflicting desires. The task is to make conscious the less conscious desires so the alliance forged does not rest solely on the patients' most superficial motivations. Illuminating their various motivations for treatment also allows the patients and prescribers to grapple with priorities and assess the adaptive value of the varying desires for treatment.

Lay the Groundwork for Good Outcomes

To effectively engage treatment resistance and the entrenched dynamics that undermine good outcomes, "many things must happen, many things must go right," as Rilke stated in the epigraph. A major goal of the maintenance phase is to use an understanding of the psychosocial dimension of pharmacotherapy and of the individual patient to optimize factors that are conducive to an desirable medication response. The other major goal of this phase is to illuminate and address, over time, the dynamic and interpersonal factors that promote treatment resistance. This is related to the psychodynamic activity of "working through" (Freud 1914/1958), in which unconsciously motivated resistances to insight are addressed by identifying unconsciously determined patterns as they interfere with the consciously agreed-upon intent of treatment. In the context of this insight, patients' resistance to change can then be explored. Whereas the working-through process of psychoanalysis focuses on depth insight and overall change, the working-through process in psychodynamic psychopharmacology is limited to those interventions that are necessary to optimize patients' use of pharmacotherapy, which may include their capacity to use less pharmacotherapy.

Optimize Factors That Support Positive Outcomes

A substantial proportion of pharmacotherapy outcomes is attributable to psychosocial aspects of pharmacotherapy, and thus the work of the maintenance phase strives to maximize these benefits. These principles hold true regardless of whether patients are naïve to treatment or have already demonstrated a degree of resistance. At this point, prescribers have in mind the many evidence-based features of the prescribing process that are associated with better outcomes, including having a patient-centered focus, expressing warmth and empathy, and supporting patients' agency. In general, prescribers attempt to optimize these factors (Table 17–1) whenever relevant. At the same time, they recognize that such population-based research glosses over individual differences. Having striven to "know who the patient is" (and not just *what* the patient is), prescribers in the maintenance phase are in a position to tailor their approach to individual patients.

> Dr. X (Chapter 5, case of Ms. C) is comfortable expressing warmth through a range of nonverbal and verbal behaviors, such as tone of voice, open body language, and empathic statements, and he does these things quite naturally. However, he came to understand that interpersonal warmth made Ms. C feel vulnerable. She voices that she does not want to feel pitied, which is how she tends to experience the kindness of others, and she hints that warmth may also feel like a seduction, evoking posttraumatic anxiety. Dr. X understands

Table 17–1. Evidence-based prescriber variables that support positive outcomes

Agreement about targets	Patient-centered focus
Autonomy support	Positive affectivity or voice tone
Belief in the treatment approach	Psychological model of illness
Empathy	Respect for treatment preferences
Good communication	Shared decision making
Investment in the patient	Warmth
Nonauthoritarian communication style	

how threatening a caregiver's kindness can feel for her and incorporates this into his psychodynamic formulation. He finds that a more neutral or even challenging stance feels more secure for Ms. C while also showing her that she interprets signs of warmth malevolently.

Keep It Appropriately Complicated and Avoid a Mind–Body Split

In the maintenance phase, when active pharmacotherapy is ongoing, prescribers maintain focus on the impact of meaning factors, resisting pulls toward reductionism. When treatment is going well, prescribers may not want to disrupt any placebo benefits by questioning whether those benefits accrue from medications or the meaning of medications. Although this strategy might make sense for treatment-naïve patients, it will likely be counterproductive for those who are treatment resistant; given these patients' history of treatment resistance, future problems may be anticipated. Ignoring the meaning of positive responses undermines the groundwork to challenge unhelpful dynamics later and runs the risk of being disempowering, particularly for treatment-resistant patients who have surrendered agency to their doctors. Instead, prescribers find opportunities to recognize the potential contribution of meaning factors to pharmacotherapy outcome:

Mr. V (see Chapter 16): I think my antidepressant is finally working.
Dr. D: Certainly, something seems to be helping. I wonder, though, how you know it is the antidepressant. I'm not saying it's not the antidepressant. It's just that I know you've also been working hard at exercising, and we've been working together to have the kind of relationship that will boost your antidepressant effects.
Mr. V: I know. It's really complicated.

Realistically, the impact of meaning factors on pharmacotherapy outcome is so significant that it is almost always impossible to know for sure the extent to which a particular outcome is driven by biomedical or psychosocial factors. To acknowledge this basic truth is, first of all, more honest. Second, it may help patients take ownership of their own self-healing capacities, fostering better outcomes. Third, it demonstrates the role of psychological and social factors when patients' defenses are not yet particularly engaged, and they are more open and receptive to learning. Waiting until there are problems means that these questions are brought up only when patients are in a more defensive stance and likely to have a harder time taking things in. It also gives a defensive patient a place from which to question the prescriber's integrity in the service of resistance.

Foster the Pharmacotherapeutic Alliance

As in the engagement phase, prescribers should be mindful to demonstrate warmth, empathy, and investment in the patient. They should engage patients in ways that emphasize and support the patients' agency. Frequently, effective prescribers deliberately foster, exploit, and ignore positive or idealizing transferences in order to boost the placebo aspects of the treatment. In psychodynamic psychopharmacology, positive transferences are similarly fostered and leveraged, but they are not generally ignored. Research suggests that placebo effects can be mobilized even when patients are aware of taking a placebo (Kaptchuk and Miller 2018; Locher et al. 2017), and acknowledging that a positive transference may be contributing to a positive outcome fosters patients' agency, as it did for Mr. V.

Attending to patients' preferences and providing opportunities for their involvement in medical decision making are crucial aspects of a solid pharmacotherapeutic alliance that may enhance treatment adherence (Woolley et al. 2010) and outcomes (Kocsis et al. 2009).

> Ms. R (see Chapter 10): What do you think about Latuda for depression? I was thinking I wanted to try that to see if it helps.
>
> Prescriber: Well, I do have some thoughts about it, but I'm curious about what makes you interested in Latuda.
>
> Ms. R: Well, someone in my support group just started it, and she says it's really helping her. It seems like a good drug.
>
> Prescriber: It's a great thought, and this might be exactly the right medication for you. Research shows it can be helpful as an add-on to your antidepressant. But the real reason it might be the right medication for you is that it's the medication that you want. As I said before, research also shows that the treatment you want will generally work better than one you don't. But it's worth noting that, in terms of the evidence, Latuda is no better than other similar medications as an adjunctive treatment for depression. It is, however, likely to be more expensive, because there is no generic yet. I can prescribe the medicine you prefer, but, given that the real difference in effectiveness has to do with your preference, you'll have to decide whether it's worth the extra cost.

Of course, such decisions must be guided by sound clinical evidence and judgment, with attention to the principle of *primum non nocere*. However, in psychiatry, one rarely finds a situation in which one medication within a class is notably more effective than other medications in that class. Patient preference, then, is a significant factor that may tip the scales in favor of a good response. Patients are also empowered when they are educated about the potential costs of their preferred treatments, both clinically and financially. Patients who are educated about potential side effects may be more likely to experience side effects (Mondaini et al. 2007; Varelmann et al. 2010), but they are also more likely to be able to tolerate those side effects if the effects have already been discussed (Bull et al. 2002) and to have a lower rate of treatment discontinuation.

Explore the Meaning of Treatment

Valuing patients' preferences does not mean that their request for new medications goes unchallenged or unexplored. Prescribers are interested in both the conscious and the unconscious motivations that underlie the request. In the earlier example, the prescriber explored Ms. R's conscious reasoning.

Consider the Meanings of Medication Changes and Requests From the Patient

Medication requests, including requests to discontinue medications, should raise questions about defensive and transference dynamics (Cabaniss 2001) (Table 17–2). For example, does a request for a medication change reflect the activation of an internal conflict for this patient?

> Ms. C (see Chapter 5), a depressed, cannabis-using young woman, is highly conflicted about her dependency both on medications and on caregivers. In his effort to formulate her treatment resistance, Dr. X relates this to her emotionally unsupportive parenting and history of sexual abuse by a teacher, for which Ms. C blames herself because of her wish for special recognition from her teacher. With this early formulation in mind, Dr. X begins to explore Ms. C's ambivalence about medications. For example, he wonders if her preference for illicit substances over prescribed medications might relate to a concern about dependency on her prescriber for something that she needs, given the ways her dependent longings have been a vehicle for hurt.
>
> When Ms. C later informs Dr. X that she wants to replace her antidepressant with an herbal supplement, Dr. X does not simply acquiesce to her request; instead, he acknowledges that her interest in herbal treatment would contribute to its potency. He is concerned about the potential for relapse, given her history of premature medication discontinuation and relapse. Although he could emphasize the recommendation that she continue antide-

Table 17–2.   Unconscious dynamics potentially underlying a request to
change or discontinue medications

Fears of facing developmentally appropriate affects leading to request for new or
more medications

Fears of dependency on medications or the prescriber leading to discontinuation
requests

Defensive wish to shift dependency from the therapist to the medications

Fears of vulnerability and a wish to control the prescriber

Complaints about medications or nonadherence representing unspoken negative
transference

Medication requests as invitations into enactment of early dynamics

pressants for 6 months after her symptoms resolve to prevent recurrence, he
anticipates that this will not address her ambivalence. Instead, he elects to explore her feelings about taking and stopping the antidepressant, which lead
to her negative feelings about dependency. He reminds her that in their first
session they had already anticipated that she might want to stop a medication
that was working because of the complex feelings it might evoke (i.e., feeling
helped and therefore dependent). Ms. C is able to acknowledge that this anxiety has led her to discontinue medications in the past, with untoward consequences. In the context of a relationship with her prescriber in which trust
has begun to develop and they have explicitly agreed to explore the psychological dimension of pharmacotherapy, Ms. C is able to acknowledge that her
desire to stop her antidepressant might be irrational, and she agrees to post-
pone discontinuation for several more months.

Similarly, medication requests may point to transference issues that are
evoked in the prescriber–patient relationship. Particularly if a framework
has been developed for looking at meaning effects in pharmacotherapy, prescribers will be in a better position to interpret the potential transference
based and irrational aspects of the request.

Several months later, Ms. C presents for her regularly scheduled pharmacotherapy appointment in a state of increased distress, having unilaterally and
abruptly discontinued her medications in the previous week. Although more
distressed than she has been for many months, she believes it is important to
stop her medications. Although they agree she has been doing much better
and that a slower taper might prevent dysphoria related to an abstinence syn-
drome, Dr. X wants to understand the renewed urgency of her wish to discontinue medications. She emphasizes that she has consistently wanted to
get off of medications but also reveals that she called her prescriber weeks
earlier with a question and learned that he was away on vacation for 2 weeks,
and she did not want to talk to the covering psychiatrist. Dr. X wonders if her
desire to get off medications so urgently relates to her distress at feeling de-

Table 17–3. Defensive functions that new prescriptions may serve for the provider

Action defenses (just do something) to defend against feeling of helplessness or hopelessness

Reaction formation with sadistic impulses disguised as heroic treatment

Medically suppressing a challenging patient to reduce the prescriber's level of agitation

Diminishing the importance of the relationship to the prescriber-therapist by shifting dependency to medications

Defensively prescribing medication to disidentify with the patient (the patient is the one taking the pill)

Utilizing medication as a defense against loss (e.g., new prescriptions at the end of a therapy)

Utilizing medications as a way of laying claim to a patient

Making a referral for consultation as an unconscious wish to be rid of the patient

---

pendent on someone who was unavailable. Ms. C can readily make this connection because it has been a subtext of several discussions, and she agrees that this might not be the optimal time and situation in which to discontinue her antidepressant. Her adherence with medications is remarkably consistent over the next 6 months, at which point she initiates a planned, cautious taper of medications. Eighteen months after her medications are terminated, she has yet not had any major depressive relapse.

Consider the Meanings of Medication Changes and Requests From the Prescriber

By the same token, when prescribers consider recommending a medication change, they should also consider whether disguised countertransference issues have been mobilized. As noted in Chapter 13, medications can serve defensive functions for prescribers (Table 17–3) by medically subduing a difficult patient, defending against feelings of helplessness, or acting as a compromise formation (Hausner 1985–1986) that ensures an ongoing symbiotic connection while still providing a safe distance from the patient. One hallmark of a defensive use of medication is that the prescriber feels better almost immediately. Although feeling better also follows competent treatment interventions, this feeling might signal an opportunity for self-reflection.

Ms. F's (see Chapters 5 and 13) defensive efforts to prevent successful antipsychotic treatment serve to preserve her child in a deathless state. Feelings of helplessness and hopelessness are evoked in her psychiatrist, causing him defensively to prescribe more aggressively in ways that prove frightening to the patient. The psychiatrist is comforted by the fact that he is prescribing treatments supported by common algorithms. It is only when he recognizes his own defenses against helplessness that he sees the unconscious logic of Ms. F's treatment resistance and can provide her the space to work through her grief enough to enter into a fuller treatment alliance with him.

Ultimately, engaging patients in an exploration of the meanings of medications, whether those medications seem to be working or not, becomes something that strengthens the fabric of the prescriber–patient relationship, making it easier to identify covert problems in that relationship and paving the way for exploring defensive and countertherapeutic aspects of pharmacotherapy.

Addressing Sources of Treatment Resistance

Predictably, the dynamic factors that have contributed to previous treatment resistance often emerge in the maintenance phase. If the engagement phase has gone well, patients understand that active treatment will involve ongoing questioning about underlying dynamics that may contribute to treatment resistance. Prescribers for treatment-resistant patients will have in mind the psychological and interpersonal characteristics known to contribute to resistance: Does the patient have a personality disorder (Bender et al. 2006; Plakun 2018; Skodol et al. 2005, 2011), immature defenses (Kronström et al. 2009), or high levels of neuroticism (Scott et al. 1995)? Is the patient sociotropic (Peselow et al. 1992), acquiescent (Fast and Fisher 1971), prone to an external locus of control (Reynaert et al. 1995), or otherwise disempowered (Hahn 1997)? Does the patient have low expectations of treatment (Aikens et al. 2005; Gaudiano and Miller 2006; Krell et al. 2004; Meyer et al. 2002; Sneed et al. 2008) or expectations of harm (Benedetti et al. 2007)?

Practitioners can operate from a population-level, evidence-based perspective that applies the available population-level evidence to individual patients who seem to fit the mold. Integrating this information into the overall diagnosis, they can consider adjustments to the treatment plan to accommodate identified sources of potential treatment resistance. The power of psychodynamic psychopharmacology is that it goes deeper than an objective-descriptive approach; its skills and techniques facilitate a highly personalized approach. Practicing this "ordinary medical psychotherapy" or "6-minute psychotherapy" (Balint 1969; Weinberg and Mintz 2018) that is integrated into routine pharmacotherapy allows personal sources of treatment resistance to be illuminated and addressed. Addressing the dynamic sources of treatment resistance hinges on prescribers' ability to blend their understanding of the patient's life history, repeating relational patterns, and core conflicts with their experience of the patient in the present.

Treatment Resistance to Medications

In cases in which treatment resistance *to* medications appears to play a major role, patients are likely in conflict in relation to some aspect of care, so addressing ambivalence will be a key aspect of treatment. Significant ambivalence will commonly manifest as nonadherence, although ambivalence may undercut medication response even when the medication is taken as recommended. Generally speaking, the major foci of patients' ambivalence include medications, the prescriber, and relinquishing symptoms.

Address Ambivalence About Medications

Ambivalence about medications forms the backdrop of almost every treatment. When patients do well with medications, it generally proves that these patients expect the benefits to outweigh the risks. However, when this ambivalence interferes with treatment, it is often due to 1) low expectations of benefit, 2) high expectations of harm, or 3) both.

The depth of the patients' ambivalence affects the types of intervention. If the ambivalence is not deep-seated, having more to do with recent negative experiences than basic expectations, then it may be sufficient to adapt the prescribing strategy (Table 17–4) without having to do much uncovering work. For patients who have low expectations of benefit, it may be beneficial to adopt a more aggressive approach that will yield faster results. For patients who have high expectations of harm, a "start-low, go-slow" strategy may avoid triggering side effects and intensifying ambivalence. Patients who have a dismissive attachment style also benefit from particularly good communication on the part of their prescriber.

Many problems with medications (e.g., nocebo responses, nonadherence) emerge in the context of feelings of powerlessness. Thus, prescribers for ambivalent patients should utilize empowering interventions. These might include addressing the patient's negative expectations straightforwardly (e.g., potential side effects), involving the patient in decision making, and eliciting patient feedback. When patients are nonadherent, prescribers might consider whether they did not sufficiently hear or respond to the patient's preferences (or concerns) about treatment. Empowering patients to play a major role in medication decisions so that they get the treatment they choose (even just choosing the dosing schedule) reduces the incidence of adverse consequences and increases the likelihood of adherence. It may be that a different medication choice will have a better outcome if its use is more under the patient's control.

The deeper the ambivalence, the more likely that aspects of it will be unconscious. Deeper ambivalence will likely have to be addressed more di-

Table 17–4.   Adjusting prescribing strategy based on expectations

	High expectation of benefit	Low expectation of benefit (dismissive style)
Low expectation of harm	No adjustment from standard prescribing process needed	More aggressive prescribing strategy to get to benefit more quickly
High expectation of harm	Slow taper to decrease likelihood of alarming side effects	Special focus on communication, framing dilemmas and involving the patient in decision making about taper

rectly (Table 17–5), beginning with the work of identifying and naming or interpreting that ambivalence. Beyond maintaining neutrality, prescribers practicing psychodynamic psychopharmacology mobilize its skills to make focal interpretations that attempt to bring such deep-seated and largely unconscious sources of ambivalence to light. Part of this focus is to help patients begin to differentiate the past and present and respond to medications as a new object and not one from the past.

In the face of significant ambivalence, prescribers strive to adopt a position, as Anna Freud (1936/1966) recommended, "at a point equidistant from the id, the ego, and the superego" (p. 28). Taking seriously that a patient has important reasons for ambivalence, the prescriber works to understand the conflicting wishes and fears that contribute to resistance while not presuming to know what the patient should choose. From a neutral, questioning stance, the prescriber then examines the discrepancies between competing wishes, goals, and values while emphasizing the role of the patient's choices and the consequences of those choices for achieving the patient's broader developmental goals. This work may also bring to light that the patient has more fundamental goals than those previously articulated (e.g., more fundamental than the goal of being able to work is the goal of being able to be loved), which may then be incorporated into the agreement on what the patient and prescriber are working on together.

In the case of Mr. B (see Chapter 5), a depressed and oppositional young man who objected to medications because his family used them to dismiss his reactions to destructive family dynamics, some groundwork was laid in the intake sessions when the patient associated taking medications with his mother "winning." At that point, the patient was already nonadherent to his medications after a brief hospitalization for a minor overdose. His child and adolescent psychiatrist expresses her expert opinion that medications may prove helpful but also recognizes that the patient has good reasons for want-

Table 17–5. Strategies for dealing with ambivalence

Strategy	Sample intervention
Identify ambivalence in the patient's treatment-resistant behaviors	"You keep saying you want to feel less depressed, but you keep stopping your antidepressants when you are feeling better. I wonder what that means about what is really important to you."
Name conscious levels of ambivalence	"It sounds like you're worried that if antidepressants work, it will mean you are weak, that you can't do it all on your own."
Offer tentative interpretations of unconscious levels of ambivalence	"This may not be right, but I get the feeling that you're reacting to me as if I want to use medications to calm you down and shut you up, kind of like your father. If that's true, I imagine that might make it a lot harder to take your medications."
Examine discrepancies among competing wishes, goals, and values	"It's obvious from everything that you say that you want to be more independent, so I'm curious about how taking or not taking your antidepressant helps you to get there. What happens when you stop taking your antidepressant? Has it been your experience that it helps you to be more independent?"
Do not presume to know what the patient should choose (unless there is imminent risk of serious harm)	"This sounds like quite a dilemma. It's really important to you to feel like you can do it on your own, but when you get depressed, it seems like it may become more difficult for you to manage on your own."
Emphasize the role of the patient's choice	"Although it sounds like medications may be helpful, I understand your reluctance. We can work together to find a way to help you get where you're trying to get. It's your choice" (within reason).

ing not to take medications. She realizes that if she pushes medications aggressively, she will likely become identified with the mother, further sparking the patient's oppositionality and provoking a negative transference. Furthermore, she believes that long-term risk can be reduced if she can form an effective alliance and work on Mr. B's ambivalence about taking medications. She suggests they continue to meet to explore this complicated issue. In subsequent sessions, she does several things to address Mr. B's ambivalence:

1. Maintains a consistent focus on his developmental goals, many of which are focused on independence but, it becomes clearer, are also focused on maintenance of self-esteem.

2. Continues to explore the patient's reasons for not wanting to take medications and interprets to him that taking medications feels like accepting the role of the identified patient in the family.
3. Highlights the consequences of medication nonadherence (recurrent depressive episodes) as they discuss the patient's history.
4. Interprets his dilemma, which is that the family dynamic has caused him to associate medications with powerlessness as opposed to associating them with an increased ability to be effective and to achieve his goals.

Her empathic recognition of his dilemma, in the absence of strong pressure to take medications, seems to make it safe for Mr. B to agree, in earnest, to try antidepressants, with his psychiatrist as a co-experimenter. Seldom is the process of working through ambivalence a "one and done" process. Practitioners of psychodynamic psychopharmacology recognize that ambivalence is deep seated, multilayered, and likely to emerge repeatedly in treatment-resistant patients.

> Mr. B is largely adherent with his medications for more than 8 months, during which time he both enrolls in community college and holds a job. Periodically, his mother still suggests that he needs more medication when they have arguments, and his doctor supports him, in their monthly or bimonthly appointments, for recognizing that vengeful impulses to stop medications could undercut his progress. However, just as he is preparing to move into an apartment, Mr. B has an argument with his mother, stops his medications, becomes depressed, and quits his job. At his next appointment, he rages about his mother and how she is ruining his life. Although she has been sympathetic with Mr. B's complicated family situation, the psychiatrist inquires about *his decision* to stop medications and quit his job. He indicates that he did not like that job anyway because he felt unfairly criticized by his boss on several occasions.
>
> Noting Mr. B's efforts to hold his mother and his boss responsible for his own self-undermining decisions, the psychiatrist suggests the possibility that Mr. B was anxious about his increasing independence, especially because repeated depressions had shaken his self-confidence in his ability to manage on his own. She speculates that although he has things to be angry about, perhaps he would rather be in a state of *hostile dependency,* in which he can avoid the emotional risks of independence while denying his resistance to greater independence. In that meeting, she also suggests that the intermittent medical psychotherapy that she has been providing might be too limited for engaging a broader and deeper struggle with separation and individuation and suggests that Mr. B also see a psychotherapist more regularly for a while.

Address Ambivalence About the Prescriber

Significant ambivalence is often associated with early disruptions in patients' caregiver and authority relationships. Transferences to treaters often mirror

Table 17–6.   Addressing transference–based resistance to
                     pharmacotherapy

Identify basic relational paradigms while obtaining a developmental history

Anticipate that these will become activated during the course of work

Listen for ways that negative transferences are creating treatment-interfering
   ambivalence

Ask: "How is the patient right?"

Name transference manifestations

Explore how transferences are impacting response to pharmacotherapy

Take responsibility for real contributions to negative transference

Explore idealizing transferences that are disempowering to the patient

transferences to medications, which also mirror basic relational patterns. Identifying and addressing negative transferences may help transform treatment resistance into treatment response (Table 17–6).

First, prescribers should be mindful of the tendency for patients and caregivers to repeat entrenched relational paradigms through the phenomenon of enactment. Recognizing that they are just as prone to unconscious acting out as their patients, prescribers should attend to feelings of discomfort and deviations from their characteristic ways of engaging patients because these may represent signs of an enactment. Except in cases in which it would significantly interfere with the work, the prescribers' effort is to avoid actualizing patients' transference fears. When a patient responds to the prescriber as a "feared negative other," it can be helpful for the prescriber to ask: "How is the patient right?"

> Mr. O (see Chapter 7) experiences Dr. A's need for him to feel better as echoing his mother's narcissistic need for him to achieve. Dr. A, in turn, experiences Mr. O's recriminations as a shameful re-creation of his own inability, as a child, to rescue his mother from depression, fueling more driven efforts to help. After identifying this dynamic in himself, Dr. A recognizes that he must find a way out of his heroic efforts to cure Mr. O so that Mr. O can believe that he is improving for himself and not for Dr. A and his narcissistic mother. Furthermore, Dr. A knows it is not enough for him to take a step back, because the rescuer/resister dynamic is well established. Rather, he has to own his part of the dynamic and offer an interpretation of this dynamic to the patient. Mr. O begins this session, as is often the case, by complaining that nothing is working and that nothing is happening except side effects.

> > Dr. A: You know, I've been thinking about how this is going, and some parts of it are starting to remind me of what you told me about you and your mother. I have a feeling that we have re-created something that is unhelpful to you, and it may be getting in the way of you getting better.

Mr. O: What do you mean? You're way different than my mother.

Dr. A: I don't mean to say that I'm exactly like her. It's more like how she pushes you to do better. I think I've reacted to your anger about not being helped enough by trying harder and harder to make you better, and that reminds me of you and your mom.

Mr. O: I mean, you are trying to help.

Dr. A: Your mom probably thinks she's helping you, too, even if it's for her own needs. I've started to feel as though maybe I've been needing you to get better even more than you need to, so it makes me like your mom.

Mr. O: Aahhh!

Dr. A: Maybe you even feel like you have to resist me, just like with your mom, so you can preserve your own separate self.

Mr. O: I don't know. I do want to feel better.

This discussion of the ways that Dr. A may have unconsciously stepped into a negative transference does not shift things immediately but becomes part of a larger discussion that unfolds over several months. Over time, Mr. O begins to recognize the limits of medication, takes small steps toward his goals, and even expresses gratitude to Dr. A for his willingness to recognize his role in an interpersonal problem, something his mother is unable to do.

When there is transference-based ambivalence about the treater, these transferences and the prescriber–patient relationship become a focus. As with transferences to medications, prescribers work with patients to expose fundamental transference expectations that are interfering with treatment so that, by working through them, patients can ally with the real prescriber and not with the problematic imaginary prescriber from the transference.

Mr. H (see Chapter 5) seems to have a therapeutic response to a trial of a selective serotonin reuptake inhibitor (SSRI) for depression and anxiety, with a marked decrease in anxiety, which seems to facilitate his engagement in therapy. However, he soon asks to discontinue his antidepressant because he is experiencing "emotional deadness." His psychiatrist initially encourages Mr. H to continue the antidepressant because he has had an otherwise positive response, and there is a possibility that the affective blunting will resolve in time. However, Mr. H's distress over this side effect escalates dramatically, and soon the medication has to be discontinued. However, at the same time, interspersed throughout his sessions, Mr. H makes comments hinting at his feeling silenced (e.g., "Oh, just put me in a cage and throw a blanket over me" and "Can't you just turn me into a zombie?").

Just after the SSRI is discontinued, his psychiatrist decodes the hidden meaning of these comments and engages this aspect of the transference. Noting that Mr H. has made these comments about feeling silenced or controlled, he wonders if Mr. H believes that the psychiatrist does not really want to hear Mr. H and is using medications to silence him, as when you put a blanket over a birdcage to stop its squawking. Mr. H resonates with this and associates it with his upbringing and the word repeatedly used by his parents when he was upset: "stifle." The psychiatrist suggests that Mr. H's emotional deadness on SSRIs could be a nocebo response to the transference-based belief that his doctor wants to stifle him. Acknowledging this possibility, Mr. H agrees to resume the SSRI, and the feeling of emotional deadness resolves.

Patients whose negative transferences spark more anger than fear may strive specifically to thwart treaters who stand in effigy of past caregivers, the true targets of the patients' wrath. To effectively confront such defeating processes (Cooperman 1989), prescribers should first consider whether they have, in fact, caused some injury, affront, or disappointment to their patient to warrant such an attack. Then, as in other cases, prescribers draw attention to the ways that patients may have displaced a fight from past caregivers onto the current one. Avenging oneself on failed caregivers can be extremely gratifying, and patients may pay a high price for the rewards of such vengeance (Cooperman 1989). Part of the ordinary medical psychotherapy of such patients involves exploring the actual costs of their vengeful solution.

It is not only negative transferences that are potentially problematic for the pharmacotherapeutic alliance. Highly idealizing transferences may also interfere with optimal outcomes. Freud recognized differential aspects of so-called positive transference: the unobjectionable part, in which more mature wishes to earn their doctor's love impel patients to put effort into treatment, and idealizing transference, which may drain patients of agency as they await cure by their almost divinely omniscient and omnipotent prescriber. When such transferences push patients into passivity, prescribers must actively confront these idealizations, emphasizing their own limitations and reliance on their patient's effort to maximize responses.

Dr. D helps Mr. V successfully stop his benzodiazepines and atypical antipsychotics. Mr. V has also been on an SSRI for 4 months at this point and is much calmer and better regulated. Dr. D has replaced the dubious diagnosis of bipolar disorder with a diagnosis of major depressive disorder complicated by borderline and narcissistic traits. Mr. V has some residual depressive symptoms, including fatigue and attentional issues, as well as some side effects, including weight gain and sexual side effects. These have not led to medication discontinuation because Mr. V has developed an apparently strong positive transference and a good working alliance with Dr. D. However, his tendency toward oversimplifying and biologizing his problems in ways that undercut his agency continues. In this session, Dr. D suggests augmentation with Wellbutrin, which might enhance Mr. V's energy, support his executive functions, and counter weight gain and sexual dysfunction. In contrast to his reported wariness about medications, Mr. V expresses optimism about this next step.

Mr. V: I'm ready. I think it's a good plan. I'm tired of just waiting for my life to happen. It's time to fix things.

Dr. D: I see this plan makes a lot of sense to you, and it does to me, too. I don't want to dampen your enthusiasm because it could help. These medications, though, as I have said, are usually not magic, even if your antidepressant is helpful. It's hard for me to know how much is your antidepressant and how much is your therapy and your life being more settled. The Wellbutrin might help, but it will probably work best if you do things like keeping up with diet and exercise.

Ambivalence About Relinquishing Symptoms

When patients are ambivalent about getting better, whether because of secondary gains of illness or defensive or communicative functions of symptoms, it is likely to be the most complicated ambivalence to maneuver (Table 17–7) because prescriber and patient easily end up in a state of misalliance. Although prescribers are invested in helping patients achieve their developmental aims, prescribers cannot sign on to the task of keeping patients in a state of illness. In most cases (except, for example, when treatment is sociopathically being used to secure secondary benefits), patients will also want to get better, so prescribers may ally with this aspect while maintaining space for the patient's significant ambivalence. To the extent that an initial alliance was formed around the task of understanding patients' subjectivity in relation to medications, prescribers may also ally in the task of further understanding patients' ambivalence about getting better.

When patients are deeply attached to symptoms or to the sick role, this often reflects a degree of disturbance that cannot be addressed adequately in 6-minute psychotherapy during occasional pharmacotherapy appointments. In such cases, it is prudent to recommend concurrent psychotherapy or combined treatment in which there can be a more sustained focus on the dynamics of the patient's treatment resistance. If the patient is already in psychotherapy, the prescriber may want to draw the therapist's attention to the dynamics of treatment resistance that emerged in the pharmacotherapy. The psychodynamic psychopharmacologist can continue, in the pharmacotherapy, to attend to signs of treatment-interfering ambivalence and bring these to the attention of the patient (and the therapist) and can continue to prescribe in a manner guided by an empathic understanding of the patient's current developmental state.

When symptoms serve to communicate something that patients are not consciously ready to acknowledge or communicate more straightforwardly, their ambivalence can be resolved if, with the help of psychotherapeutic interventions, they can become aware of these suppressed feelings and capable of putting them into words so that they can be addressed more directly.

Table 17–7. Addressing ambivalence about relinquishing symptoms

Attempt to identify such ambivalence early before misalliance is enacted

Ally with the part of the patient that is invested in recovery

Consider referral for psychotherapy

Help translate communicative functions of symptoms

Respect defensive functions of symptoms, attempting to remain neutral

Identify and name secondary gains that could promote treatment resistance

Highlight discrepancies between attachment to symptoms and developmental goals

---

Ms. R (see Chapter 10) appears to be doing much better. She initially presented for significant depression in the context of the stresses of motherhood and an unconscious competition with her infant daughter for her husband's attention. With therapy, a modest dosage of an antidepressant, and augmentation with an atypical neuroleptic, the neurovegetative symptoms of her depression are substantially but not completely resolved, and she has been able to return to work. However, she calls her psychiatrist to schedule an appointment because of worsening symptoms over the previous week.

Attentive to the meaning of symptomatic changes, her psychiatrist asks her thoughts about her proximal stressors. Ms. R discusses several stressors at home and work and several times notes that her therapist had taken a vacation just as these stresses were presenting. At one point, she also seems to make a snide remark about her beloved therapist's time away. The psychiatrist observes that Ms. R seems angry at her therapist. Ms. R replies that she is not angry but is frustrated that her therapist chose that particular time to go on vacation, when she had just moved to the float team in the hospital and her husband had just had a promotion that was taking more of his time. The psychiatrist asks if Ms. R has expressed these frustrations to her therapist and learns that she has not. Acknowledging both that depression is sometimes a manifestation of anger turned inward and that she has had increased depression for less than 2 weeks, the psychiatrist reviews the treatment options and suggests Ms. R first discuss her frustration with the therapist to see if this helps her feel better. She offers a back-up plan of increasing Ms. R's antidepressant, which is currently at a moderate dosage; she offers to send the prescription to the pharmacy if Ms. R calls next week to say she still needs it. The psychiatrist also tells Ms. R that she would like to call the therapist herself.

In this intervention, the psychiatrist does several things to introduce meaning, to support Ms. R's self-understanding and agency, and to ultimately prevent medications from being prescribed unnecessarily. She 1) holds in mind Ms. R's history of and sensitivity to abandonment; 2) investigates the deeper meanings of new or increased symptoms; 3) interprets the possible meaning of worsening symptoms (expressing symptomatically the interpersonal anger or frustration that Ms. R cannot put into words); 4) suggests ways that the patient may, through her own effort, obtain some mastery over the symptoms; and 5) in sending her away without a new prescription, reminds Ms. R that the resource (and the psychiatrist) is still at her disposal, so as to not prompt further abandonment anxieties. The psychiatrist also calls the therapist to avoid any potential splitting because Ms. R has offered veiled criticisms of her therapist, and the psychiatrist has offered an interpretation relevant to Ms. R's request for medications. (For a fuller exposition of techniques in split treatment, please see Chapter 18.) Ms. R does not call back, and at their next regularly scheduled appointment, she informs the psychiatrist that "it was just a blip" and that things seemed to resolve once she was able to express her displeasure about the therapist's vacation, to which the therapist responded empathically and respectfully.

When symptoms serve important defensive functions, patients are likely to remain highly ambivalent about relinquishing them until the patients are able to find substitute gratifications or develop alternate coping strategies. This developmental process takes time, so prescribers should be prepared that, in such cases, laying the groundwork for successful treatment may take months or longer.

> Ms. F's resistance to effective treatment appears to be driven in large measure by the defense of psychotic restitution, allowing her deceased child to remain alive (or possibly alive) in her psychotic fantasy. Her prescriber, in coming to a formulation of her treatment resistance, is able to contain his frustration and provide a more empathic and unobtrusive (but not optimally effective) pharmacological support. Meanwhile, in her therapy, she works on her grief. After 6–8 months, Ms. F has done enough grief work that she can tolerate a more effective medication, no longer gripped by the conviction that it will cause her to attempt suicide. She starts clozapine, to good effect. She becomes better organized and more related, and her delusions resolve. However, in what is possibly an optimal outcome for the patient, she never loses the hallucinated voice of her dead child.

When the sick role offers significant gratification, treatment can be truly challenging, particularly if the likely rewards of health are relatively meager compared with the rewards of the sick role. Most frequently, such patients will be unaware (or only dimly aware) that they are choosing illness and its covert gratifications over health. Their readiness to change is cultivated first by helping them see how they may be choosing illness over health. Like patients who are gratified by the opportunity to vengefully thwart caregivers, their attention must be drawn to the actual costs of this solution, which are often considerable. These patients, who have surrendered many mature satisfactions, may derive much comfort from their relationship with their psychiatric caregivers. The unobjectionable part of this positive transference may predispose them to strive to be good for their doctor and become another motivation for them to consider giving up the gratifications of their illness. For this reason, the quality of the prescriber–patient relationship is critical.

In some cases, patients may also be ambivalent regarding the absence of symptoms while being largely invested in recovery. In this case, the process of getting better provokes their anxiety rather than the loss of particular gratifications of illness. This is sometimes the case with patients who have experienced major breakdowns associated with feelings of well-being, such as occurs in mania. Such patients may become highly suspicious of feelings of well-being, which are now associated with a frightening loss of control. They may intentionally or unconsciously dismantle happy feelings and cultivate states of low-grade depression out of a fear that good feelings are harbingers of mania. Focal psychotherapeutic work may help these patients differentiate healthy feelings of well-being from signs of mania so that they do not have to resist the antidepressant aspects of pharmacotherapy.

Treatment Resistance From Medication

When patients describe medications as effective for target symptoms yet do not appear over time to improve functionally, prescribers should consider whether some countertherapeutic use of treatment or meaning of treatment is contributing to treatment resistance (Table 17–8). In such cases, prescribers are made into unwitting accomplices in a perverse use of treatment. Often, prescribers become aware of this through a countertransference experience of unease that can function as a sign of treatment resistance from medication. In psychodynamic psychopharmacology, this unease signals that the prescriber must attend to countertransference reactions (see Chapters 7 and 13) and consider what information this reaction provides about unconscious aspects of the treatment.

Treatment resistance from medications (see Chapter 6) and treatment resistance to medications (see Chapter 5) are not mutually exclusive. Patients with immature defenses, significant defensive needs, significant interpersonal dysfunction, and a disordered relationship with their own agency are more likely to have a complicated relationship with pharmacotherapy in which treatment may both be resisted and turned defensively to serve countertherapeutic ends. These patients are also likely to demonstrate a greater degree of treatment resistance.

When prescribers assess patients as having some degree of treatment resistance *from* medications, they may experience an impulse to immediately deprescribe to limit the harm done by medications. However, the work of psychodynamic psychopharmacology is aimed at supporting a developmental process, the end result of which will be the patient's increased capacity to use pharmacotherapy in a healthy and effective way. Abrupt and unilateral

Table 17–8.   Addressing treatment resistance *from* medications

Attend to countertransference clues that treatment is contributing to chronicity

Resist immediate impulse to deprescribe unless there is a threat of medical harm

Question medicalized understandings that undercut hopefulness and agency

Explore origins of deauthorizing assumptions regarding pharmacotherapy

Continue to express realistic humility about what medications alone can accomplish

Differentiate "problems of illness" from "problems of living"; find meaning in feelings

Encourage help seeking when medications have come to replace people

Focus on coping skills when patients have become deskilled by overreliance on medication

Taper at a rate that allows patients to adjust to and cope with new levels of feeling

deprescribing, particularly in the absence of a solid pharmacotherapeutic alliance, may solve the problem in the short term but may undercut the ability to use the pharmacotherapeutic alliance to promote healthy change and to deepen the patient's defensive attachment to medications. In such cases, when iatrogenic effects of pharmacotherapy emerge from the psychosocial dimension of treatment, these problems are likely best addressed by interventions at that same level. Rarely, except in cases in which patients are using medications in an acutely medically harmful way (e.g., as an intoxicant or parasuicidally), is there a need for abrupt medication discontinuation, particularly if patients are attached to their regimen.

When treatment causes harm and contributes to patients' treatment resistance, this can take several forms that call for different technical interventions. Harm that originates from the meaning of medications may remain at the meaning level, adversely affecting patients primarily at the ideational level (e.g., creating harmful ways of understanding the self). Alternately, medications can take on defensive functions that impair patients' self-understanding and personal agency, thus helping them remain stuck. Pharmacotherapy can also substitute for adaptive capacities and emotional coping in ways that keep patients from developing more mature coping skills.

Adverse Effects on Identity and Self-Concept

Patients may internalize pharmacotherapy and its meanings into personal identity in ways that prove developmentally harmful. Medications may become a concrete symbol that patients are bad, crazy, or intolerable to others. Ingesting these ideas every day in the form of medications may certainly interfere with these patients' capacity to achieve their full potential. Biogenic explanations (Kemp et al. 2014) may prove particularly disabling, creating helplessness and hopelessness that undercut medication efforts and impair patients' sense of personal agency (i.e., creating negative mood-regulation expectancies), worsening outcomes. To the extent that these meaning-based adverse consequences are derived largely from misunderstandings, continued psychoeducation may be sufficient to alleviate this source of treatment resistance from medications.

> Dr. X tries, when negotiating new antidepressants, to emphasize that there are both psychological and biological contributions to depression and that there are things that the patient can also do to foster recovery, such as exercise, spend time in nature, and engage in pleasurable and healthy activities. Frequently, Dr. X also highlights how reliance on medications alone to solve complex problems may create complacency.

When patients have internalized noxious ideas about medications, they have a reason for doing so. If these ideas are not serving a defensive function, they may have been internalized from people who have influence over the patient, such as a prescriber who caused inadvertent harm by offering overly biomedical explanations or family members for whom these ideas serve a defensive function (e.g., allowing the "bad" or the "crazy" to be localized in the person taking the pill). In such cases, mere psychoeducation may be inadequate to counter projective identifications. Interventions would have to address the larger family system and might include psychoeducation of the family, family therapy to address identified patient dynamics, or individual psychotherapeutic work to assist patients in differentiating themselves from their family so as to be less vulnerable to such projections.

Treatment as a Defense

When treatment functions as a symptom, representing a defensive compromise, patients often consciously experience specific treatments as helpful and may become quite attached to them. Meanwhile, they appear to be in a process of chronification, in which diagnoses, treatment, or medications take a prominent role in their lives. However, in such cases, feelings are increasingly confused with symptoms, and a sense of personal agency is supplanted with medical understanding and biomedical controls. Because such misuses of treatment are typically unconscious, prescribers must be attentive to such covert dynamics. Often, prescribers experience these patients as surrendering agency to the treatment, perhaps by developing a biologized view of themselves or seeking medical solutions for feelings that a healthier person would recognize as normative.

Sir William Osler observed that the desire to take medication is a primary characteristic that distinguishes humans from animals, although the desire for care is often the driving factor. Particularly in the context of early failures in caregiving and current life circumstances, patients may regress to states of infantile dependency. Seeking to gratify early longings for inexhaustible and nearly all-powerful care, such patients approach treatment as though the receipt of care is the goal of treatment, not recovery. Although the value these patients place on treatment may initially be gratifying, it often becomes noxious when prescribers experience the difference between the enormity of their patient's desire for perfect care and their own meager resources. In addition, prescribers may notice that their patient is resisting effective care to receive some gratification from treatment. Occasionally, or more frequently in busy and stressed systems, hateful countertransferences are veiled by policies and procedures intended to disabuse patients of any notion that they will receive emotionally gratifying psychiatric care. Although this may spare treaters, it seldom helps patients to recover.

The first bit of work prescribers do when they encounter such a regressive use of care is to become aware of, contain, and ultimately use countertransference; avoid overpromising so as not to collude with expectations of omnipotent care; and develop a dynamic formulation of the nature of the resistance. The last, informed by the countertransference, allows prescribers empathically to begin addressing the dynamics underlying patients' treatment resistance and serves as a reminder that no matter how countertherapeutic patients' use of medications appears to be, patients are always trying to solve some important developmental challenge. If anything, it is helpful to meet with these patients more often rather than less, at least for a time. During these meetings, appropriate limits should be set, the limits of what medications can do in the absence of effort from the patient should be emphasized with realistic humility, and an effort to start interpreting—as Havens (1968) said, "from not too great a distance" (p. 47)—the early roots of a transferential hunger for pharmacological care should be made so it can be grappled with consciously rather than enacted unconsciously.

> Ms. G (see Chapter 5) has experienced many early abandonments and losses and is afraid that if she gets better she will lose her psychiatrist as well. She decompensates following his suggestion that some of her medications may no longer be necessary. This particular decompensation alerts her psychiatrist to ways that she might be motivated to remain ill to justify her ongoing connection to him. In response, he decides to offer the following hypothesis.
>
> Psychiatrist: Do you think I might have scared you when I said I didn't think you needed the Seroquel anymore?
> Ms. G: Yeah. What if I start getting panic again?
> Psychiatrist: Well, of course, we would deal with it…but I was also thinking that you've had so much loss and wondering if you worried that you might lose me if you got better.

Ms. G: You're the best doctor I've ever had.

Psychiatrist: I think maybe that you got so anxious that your anxiety went way up. And I think, too, that maybe, on some level, you could be scared to get better because you are scared of losing your supports, like me.

Ms. G: You know I want to get better.

Psychiatrist: I know you do, but I also know people are complicated and can have lots of different feelings and that one of the things that helps you feel better is having stable people in your life.

Ms. G: That's true.

Psychiatrist: If you are scared about that, I can say that there is no reason for us to meet less often if you are on less medication.

In this interaction, the psychiatrist does a number of things to address the ways that illness serves as a defense against loss. He 1) considers the role of Ms. G's developmental history in her relation to illness; 2) ascertains that one of her primary, albeit unspoken, and understandable goals is to avoid further experiences of loss; 3) interprets her decompensation as a possible attachment to illness intended to prevent loss; 4) empathically addresses Ms. G's anxiety; and 5) works to restore an alliance in relation to healthy and mutually agreed-upon goals. At the end of that session, they agree on a reduction in Seroquel, and the psychiatrist emphasizes that he would like to see Ms. G more frequently while medication changes are being made, recognizing that she equates losing medication with losing her doctor.

Treatment resistance may emerge when patients use biomedical explanations defensively to disavow aspects of the self, avoid self-knowledge, and escape unpleasant but developmentally appropriate feelings by medicalizing them. Such patients experience some relief from treatment but impair their agency, adaptability, and ability to use emotions in the process. Changing medications may bring temporary relief because such action, together with prescribers' unwitting collusion, helps fortify their defense. Unfortunately, because it does not solve the underlying issues, treatment often becomes a perpetual pursuit of treating bad feelings with more and more medications. Again, having an empathic formulation regarding the struggles that spark such a defense allows prescribers first to contain their own impulsive actions and to lean on the agreement to explore the meaning of medication requests, loss of response, or new complaints.

Paying close attention to the events (internal and external) leading up to distressing new "symptoms," prescribers work with patients to differentiate symptoms and feelings, or "problems of illness" versus "problems of living" (B. Belnap, personal communication, 2010) before deciding to medicate. However, this is not just a short-term solution to potentially inappropriate or unnecessary prescribing. Integrating such ordinary medical psychotherapy into patients' pharmacological care can, over time, help reorient these patients to the signal function of their affects so they can begin to establish (or reestablish) affect competence and a capacity to mentalize (Jurist 2010).

> Ms. T (see Chapter 11) arrives at her prescriber's office in her residential program stating that she needs to discontinue gabapentin because it is making her angry. There is much to understand about how she experiences medications as responsible for her emotional state. Her depression and anxiety (and timidity) appear to improve as a consequence of psychotherapy or pharmacotherapy with an SSRI plus a GABAergic anticonvulsant, or both, so her dysphoria is a notable shift. Her psychiatrist, as a member of her treatment team, knows that her family has just precipitously withdrawn support for her treatment. He has already established, over months of work, that he would likely be interested in the meanings of clinical changes and requests for changes to the medication regimen. Even without information related to her family context, he would likely have questioned her attribution of anger to her medications.

> Psychiatrist: You know, I tend to think of feelings as having some kind of meaning. I mean, hundreds of thousands of years have gone into producing our emotions, which are a kind of sense organ that gives us information to help us navigate the social world. Of course, that can go awry and cause sickness, but it's all very complicated. It makes me curious to know how you *know* it's the gabapentin that made you angry.
>
> Ms. T: Well, it kind of just came out of nowhere. There is no reason for me to be angry. The last medication change that I had was the gabapentin [2.5 months earlier].
>
> Psychiatrist: Well, before we rush to make that feeling go away, I wonder if we could first see if there's something that feeling is trying to tell us.
>
> Ms. T: Okay.
>
> Psychiatrist: Could you tell me a little bit more about that feeling, about what it was like?
>
> Ms. T: I just felt angry on Sunday, like I wanted to smash something.
>
> Psychiatrist: To smash something?
>
> Ms. T: Yeah, I don't know what, though.
>
> Psychiatrist: Something that was yours? Something that was ours?
>
> Ms. T: I wanted to throw something…my phone, maybe. But then I wanted to hit myself on the head. I thought I was going to, but I didn't. I didn't do anything. That's when I decided to call you.
>
> Psychiatrist: You wanted that feeling to go away. It was bad. So bad that you wanted to beat your head.
>
> Ms. T: Yeah. I'm not usually an angry person.
>
> Psychiatrist: And you feel like it just came out of the blue?
>
> Ms. T: I mean, I think I was already in a bad mood. I was just cranky all weekend. That's just not me.
>
> Psychiatrist: Do you remember what was going on when you first noticed that you were angry?

Ms. T: I feel like I just woke up that way…Saturday.

Psychiatrist: So, it makes me wonder what was happening in your life. Were there any interactions with anyone that stand out?

Ms. T: I did talk to my folks on Friday night. They let me know that there wasn't money anymore [for treatment].

Psychiatrist: Aaah. Can I ask what that was like?

Ms. T: I don't know. I wasn't really expecting it, but they've been really supportive. I can't complain.

Psychiatrist: You can't complain? Do you know about what?

Ms. T: I don't know. I kind of wish I had a little more warning.

Psychiatrist: So, this all makes me wonder if your anger was telling you something important…maybe about how you feel about the ending of your treatment. But, like you say, you can't complain, so it seems like a tough spot.

Ms. T: Uh-huh.

Psychiatrist: It really makes me wonder if it's the gabapentin, especially because you've been on it for a few months already with no problems. I'm worried that if we decide it's the gabapentin before we really understand, it might make it harder for you to make sense of your feelings. Do you think it would be okay if we held off on making a change until you've a chance to talk to your therapist about this? If, after talking it through, it still seems the gabapentin is causing problems, just let me know.

Ms. T brings this to her therapist (whom her psychiatrist also contacts). Over the next 2 weeks it becomes clearer that Ms. T is facing a family culture that does not tolerate anger, especially her anger. She even speculates that her growing aliveness might be one of the reasons her treatment resources were ended so precipitously. Her psychiatrist's refusal to immediately collude with a dynamic that pathologized Ms. T's emotions offers an opportunity for her to see, in the here and now, how things that she could not say were being experienced (typically somatically), medicalized, and discarded as meaningless.

When Medications Replace People

As noted in Chapter 6, patients may use medications as part of a counterdependent strategy in which, instead of turning to people for comfort, they turn to medications, which function as a kind of transitional object. This creates a vicious circle whereby their world is increasingly depopulated, increasing their dysphoria and need for medication to quell the distress of isolation.

Abrupt and unilateral deprescribing runs the risk of deepening patients' conviction that people are unreliable, particularly if done early in the therapeutic relationship. At the same time, prescribers should not collude with a defense that is likely to contribute to chronification. Once this countertherapeutic use of medications is identified and becomes a focus of exploration, prescribers may negotiate a plan for the patient to forestall use of as-needed medications until they first try other coping strategies, including seeking support from others. For patients who have dismissive attachments or a very low tolerance for frustration, this work may be facilitated by involving them in support-rich environments, including residential and intensive outpatient programs, group therapy, and forms of individual therapy with high levels of therapist availability. For such patients, reduced or discontinued medications should not lead, at least initially, to reduced attention from the doctor.

When Medications Substitute for Ego Functions

Many patients who rely heavily on medications to manage transient states of distress will acquire significant deficits in their capacity to regulate affect, particularly when medicated from an early age or prescribed medications in part to address preexisting ego deficits. These patients are easily overcome by intense, unmanageable anxiety and other dysphoric states. They are also caught in a vicious circle in which ignoring the signal functions of their distress leaves them unable to effectively address real-world sources of anxiety. For such patients, developmentally focused prescribing aims toward deprescribing (at least those medications being used to substitute for internal controls). In most cases, this is a slow process. However, as small decreases allow patients, over time, to develop their coping capacity, they will be less prone to feeling overwhelmed.

For patients who derive significant secondary gains from the sick role, tending to the alliance is especially important. Often, they are unambivalently attached to their medications and highly motivated to maintain access to and control over these medications, for which they feel a pressing need when in states of distress. The dilemma they face may be identified and discussed ahead of any actual medication changes, allowing time for a treatment alliance to deepen. Again, because patients are typically unaware of the ways their use of medications is interfering with their development, the early work is spent examining the ways they are actually using their medications.

The primary aims of this initial work are to identify unconscious sources of ambivalence, bring ambivalence to conscious awareness, and respect patients' dilemmas. At the same time, prescribers question defensive aspects of hopelessness and helplessness that can cause patients to surrender their agency and self-efficacy to the treatment. In this way, hope may be restored, allowing patients to get back on the developmental trajectory of learning to manage their feelings. Like patients who have so defensively medicalized themselves that they no longer have feelings, patients who have substituted medications for internal controls may benefit from close attention to their "symptoms." By exploring the antecedents of dysphoric states (that patients report as symptoms) and the fears and conflicts evoked, patients may become reacquainted with their feeling life and reminded that there is a sense to their feelings that is to be understood and respected.

As Freud (1911/1958) noted, people will never willingly surrender a gratification without some form of compensation. Thus, addressing patients' treatment-interfering ambivalence often involves understanding what might constitute compensation. Certainly, the promise of a more fulfilling life is one potential source of compensation. However, many of these patients cannot imagine better things are possible. They may benefit from added support while they grapple with difficult feelings they previously strove to suppress with medications. Although the added support that comes with psychotherapeutic attention to their emotional life may be sufficient, increased availability of the prescriber (e.g., meeting bimonthly or monthly instead of every 3 months) during times of emotional strain may also serve as compensation for the medications being given up. As for those who have replaced people with medications, more regular supports, including psychotherapies aimed at mentalizing and increasing affect tolerance, as well as intensive outpatient programs or residential treatment, may provide them with enough support that they can bear to give up their unhelpful attachment to medications.

Lacking healthy emotional controls, these patients are prone to experiencing intense and frightening affect states. Control struggles often manifest in treatment as patients desperately work to establish equilibrium. Although it is easy to become embroiled in power struggles, better long-term outcomes may be achieved if prescribers can give their patients some control of the deprescribing process while working consistently toward increasing the patients' capacity to self-regulate. Patients should be given choices regarding the rate of medication taper and as-needed dosing schedules or be offered less destructive replacements. Regular medications may be renegotiated to as-needed instead of regular dosing, giving patients control over their rate of taper. When patients encounter stressful situations, they may wish to resume higher dosages. Prescribers then will have to decide whether to hold the line over hard-won gains or support patients' requests, keeping in mind that if patients believe their prescriber will respect their wishes during times of particular distress, they may find it easier to risk accelerated deprescribing in the future. These decisions may be shaped by the prescribers' assessment of these patients' characterological ego strengths and usable superego (see Chapter 9).

> In the treatment of Mr. K (see Chapter 6), the work of restoring his sense of self-efficacy and reducing overreliance on medications takes the better part of a year because treatment has to address 1) a deeply ingrained family dynamic that wants to strip his symptoms of meaning and reduce them to mere aberrant biology, 2) Mr. K's true dread over the possibility of loss of control

and becoming more solidly identified as the bad one, and 3) real and significant deficits in affective coping skills that have come about as a consequence of relying on medications to deal with almost all bad feelings.

In the first or second session, the prescriber exclaims: "Wow, it looks like someone really wants to control you" in response to the number of sedating medications in Mr. K's regimen. This effort to make meaning of the medication regimen is not acknowledged in the moment; however, at a later point, Mr. K remembers this remark, and it becomes one of the reasons he is willing to experience the distress of increasing agency.

Before that, however, there are several months of preparatory work in which Mr. K comes to understand that medication is *potentially* harmful, which allows him to join his prescriber in the decision to explore reducing medication. This is followed by a long process of experimenting with minor decreases in medications as encouraged by the prescriber, who thinks Mr. K's level of sedation interferes with his ability to engage fully in residential treatment. The patient visits his home after the first reduction of an antipsychotic, and his family calls to report that he is becoming manic. This is curious, because he has shown no evidence of mania in the residential setting. Mr. K agrees with his family's assessment.

Over time, each medication reduction is followed by anxious fears of losing control and feelings of being overwhelmed. The family continues to report episodes of mania when he is on home visits, but as the episodes and their precipitants are explored, it becomes clear first to the prescriber and then to Mr. K that he is angry and not manic. Coming to see this and understanding that his developmentally appropriate anger has been pathologized to serve a larger family dynamic, Mr. K becomes more resolved to take as few medications as needed.

Regardless of prescribers' specific medical decisions, they continuously consider how countertransferences may be impacting these decisions. Does giving the patient more control serve, for example, the prescriber's conflict avoidance? Beyond self-reflection, prescribers can check themselves by assessing whether progress is actually being made.

Medication as Fetish

If patients are making little progress toward deprescribing and a healthier relationship with pharmacotherapy, prescribers should consider whether the medication has been fetishized. In this case, access to and control over the medication are the patient's overarching concern, and any appearance of working toward deprescribing is likely an effort to forestall action and control the prescriber. Prescribers cannot indefinitely continue to prescribe a medication that does more harm than good, however, in the absence of evidence that there is movement toward a healthier solution. This is one case in which prescribers may unilaterally decide to deprescribe, holding in mind that patients may leave treatment to maintain access to their chosen substance.

Biomedically Mediated Harm

Although in most cases treatment resistance *from* medication unfolds at the level of meaning, developmental harm may, at times, be caused by biological effects of the medication. This was the case with Mr. K, who, in response to a powerful family defense, has been maintained on highly sedating medications since childhood, markedly impairing both his cognitive and emotional development. Such patients will not achieve optimal function until the impairing medications are reduced or discontinued. Deprescribing, however, may not be urgent and may be accomplished with less pain and greater long-term success if carefully negotiated with the patient and titrated to match the patient's emerging capacities for self-regulation.

> Mr. K's prescriber takes a stronger position than normal, stressing that they have to explore medication reduction because he believes he is causing Mr. K harm by prescribing them. Mr. K eventually comes to see his own struggles more as problems of living (anger over a pathologizing family dynamic) than as problems of illness. Psychiatric issues remain to be addressed, including both his neurodevelopmental deficits in executive functioning and the developmental deficits that have evolved because he has almost always used medications to manage states of dysphoric arousal and thus has underdeveloped coping skills.
>
> Each reduction in medication is accompanied by increased anxiety because Mr. K encounters a new level of feeling that he is not quite ready to bear. To discontinue medications too quickly may also cause unnecessary harm. Continued work to name his feelings and put them in a meaningful context makes them easier to bear (as opposed to experiencing them as random, senseless, and unfair biological afflictions). Tapering at a rate that is tolerable, together with a focus on developing healthier affective coping, allows Mr. K to feel in control of the process and of himself as he develops skills that have been supplanted by medications.

Working With Countertransference

As the doctor–patient relationship unfolds, subtle hurts and disappointments will accumulate, negative transferences are sparked, interpersonal defenses are mobilized, and primitive modes of defense and communication (splitting and projective identification) project the patient's (and doctor's) inner world into the outer world. Under these circumstances, prescribers are more likely to be induced into enactments and other forms of irrationality. As detailed in Chapter 13, prescribers should remain open to the potential for their own irrationality. To manage this irrationality, they can employ strategies such as asking "How is the patient right?" when patients complain or act defensively, attempting to use countertransference reactions as a source of understanding of the patient, taking responsibility for misalliance when appropriate, and consulting with colleagues and using a psychodynamic formulation to reestablish balance.

Key Points

- Attending to an evidence-based pharmacotherapy process (e.g., showing warmth and empathy, attending to the alliance, integrating patient preferences into medical decision making) may prevent the emergence or worsening of treatment resistance.

- Prescribers should listen for and address or interpret disempowering assumptions that patients attach to medications in the process of routine pharmacotherapy.

- Changes in clinical status should not be attributed reflexively to medications and should prompt questions about psychological or interpersonal factors that are contributing, positively or negatively, to outcomes.

- Requests for medication changes or consultations are occasions to reflect on whether there are unrecognized strains in the prescriber–patient alliance.

- Interventions should aim consistently to emphasize the role that patients' agency has, both manifestly and unconsciously, in their own recovery.

References

Aikens JE, Kroenke K, Swindle RW, et al: Nine-month predictors and outcomes of SSRI antidepressant continuation in primary care. Gen Hosp Psychiatry 27(4):229–236, 2005 15993253

Balint E: The possibilities of patient-centered medicine. J R Coll Gen Pract 17(82):269–276, 1969 5770926

Bender DS, Skodol AE, Pagano ME, et al: Prospective assessment of treatment use by patients with personality disorders. Psychiatr Serv 57(2):254–257, 2006 16452705

Benedetti F, Lanotte M, Lopiano L, et al: When words are painful: unraveling the mechanisms of the nocebo effect. Neuroscience 147(2):260–271, 2007 17379417

Bull SA, Hu XH, Hunkeler EM, et al: Discontinuation of use and switching of antidepressants: influence of patient-physician communication. JAMA 288(11):1403–1409, 2002 12234237

Cabaniss DL: Beyond dualism: psychoanalysis and medication in the 21st century. Bull Menninger Clin 65(2):160–170, 2001 11407140

Cooperman MC: Defeating processes in psychotherapy, in Psychoanalysis and Psychosis. Edited by Silver AS. Madison, CT, International Universities Press, 1989, pp 339–357

Fast GJ, Fisher S: The role of body attitudes and acquiescence in epinephrine and placebo effects. Psychosom Med 33(1):63–84, 1971 5100735

Freud A: The ego and the mechanisms of defense (1936), in The Writings of Anna Freud, Vol 2. New York, International Universities Press, 1966

Freud S: Formulations on the two principles of mental functioning (1911), in Standard Edition of the Complete Psychological Works of Sigmund Freud, Vol 12. Translated and edited by Strachey J. London, Hogarth, 1958, pp 218–226

Freud S: On beginning the treatment (further recommendations on the technique of psycho-analysis I) (1913), in Standard Edition of the Complete Psychological Works of Sigmund Freud, Vol 12. Translated and edited by Strachey J. London, Hogarth, 1958, pp 121–144

Freud S: Remembering, repeating and working-through (further recommendations on the technique of psycho-analysis II) (1914), in Standard Edition of the Complete Psychological Works of Sigmund Freud, Vol 12. Translated and edited by Strachey J. London, Hogarth, 1958, pp 145–156

Gaudiano BA, Miller IW: Patients' expectancies, the alliance in pharmacotherapy, and treatment outcomes in bipolar disorder. J Consult Clin Psychol 74(4):671–676, 2006 16881774

Hahn RA: The nocebo phenomenon: scope and foundations, in The Placebo Effect: An Interdisciplinary Exploration. Edited by Harrington A. Cambridge, MA, Harvard University Press, 1997, pp 56–76

Hausner R: Medication and transitional phenomena. Int J Psychoanal Psychother 11:375–407, 1985–1986 4086185

Havens LL: Some difficulties in giving schizophrenic and borderline patients medication. Psychiatry 31(1):44–50, 1968 5637281

Jurist E: Mentalizing minds. Psychoanalytic Inquiry 30(4):289–300, 2010

Kaptchuk TJ, Miller FG: Open label placebo: can honestly prescribed placebos evoke meaningful therapeutic benefits? BMJ 363:k3889, 2018 30279235

Kemp JJ, Lickel JJ, Deacon BJ: Effects of a chemical imbalance causal explanation on individuals' perceptions of their depressive symptoms. Behav Res Ther 56:47–52, 2014 24657311

Kocsis JH, Leon AC, Markowitz JC, et al: Patient preference as a moderator of outcome for chronic forms of major depressive disorder treated with nefazodone, cognitive behavioral analysis system of psychotherapy, or their combination. J Clin Psychiatry 70(3):354–361, 2009 19192474

Krell HV, Leuchter AF, Morgan M, et al: Subject expectations of treatment effectiveness and outcome of treatment with an experimental antidepressant. J Clin Psychiatry 65(9):1174–1179, 2004 15367043

Kronström K, Salminen JK, Hietala J, et al: Does defense style or psychological mindedness predict treatment response in major depression? Depress Anxiety 26(7):689–695, 2009 19496102

Locher C, Frey Nascimento A, Kirsch I, et al: Is the rationale more important than deception? A randomized controlled trial of open-label placebo analgesia. Pain 158(12):2320–2328, 2017 28708766

Meyer B, Pilkonis PA, Krupnick JL, et al: Treatment expectancies, patient alliance, and outcome: further analyses from the National Institute of Mental Health Treatment of Depression Collaborative Research Program. J Consult Clin Psychol 70(4):1051–1055, 2002 12182269

Mondaini N, Gontero P, Giubilei G, et al: Finasteride 5 mg and sexual side effects: how many of these are related to a nocebo phenomenon? J Sex Med 4(6):1708–1712, 2007 17655657

Peselow ED, Robins CJ, Sanfilipo MP, et al: Sociotropy and autonomy: relationship to antidepressant drug treatment response and endogenous-nonendogenous dichotomy. J Abnorm Psychol 101(3):479–486, 1992 1386856

Plakun EM: Psychodynamic psychiatry, the biopsychosocial model, and the difficult patient. Psychiatr Clin North Am 34(2):237–248, 2018

Reynaert C, Janne P, Vause M, et al: Clinical trials of antidepressants: the hidden face: where locus of control appears to play a key role in depression outcome. Psychopharmacology (Berl) 119(4):449–454, 1995 7480525

Scott J, Williams JM, Brittlebank A, et al: The relationship between premorbid neuroticism, cognitive dysfunction and persistence of depression: a 1-year follow-up. J Affect Disord 33(3):167–172, 1995 7790668

Skodol AE, Gunderson JG, Shea MT, et al: The Collaborative Longitudinal Personality Disorders Study (CLPS): overview and implications. J Pers Disord 19(5):487–504, 2005 16274278

Skodol AE, Grilo CM, Keyes KM, et al: Relationship of personality disorders to the course of major depressive disorder in a nationally representative sample. Am J Psychiatry 168(3):257–264, 2011 21245088

Sneed JR, Rutherford BR, Rindskopf D, et al: Design makes a difference: a meta-analysis of antidepressant response rates in placebo-controlled versus comparator trials in late-life depression. Am J Geriatr Psychiatry 16(1):65–73, 2008 17998306

Varelmann D, Pancaro C, Cappiello EC, et al: Nocebo-induced hyperalgesia during local anesthetic injection. Anesth Analg 110(3):868–870, 2010 20042440

Weinberg E, Mintz D: The overall diagnosis: psychodynamic psychiatry, six-minute psychotherapy, and patient-centered care. Psychiatr Clin North Am 41(2):263–275, 2018 29739525

Woolley SB, Fredman L, Goethe JW, et al: Hospital patients' perceptions during treatment and early discontinuation of serotonin selective reuptake inhibitor antidepressants. J Clin Psychopharmacol 30(6):716–719, 2010 21105288

CHAPTER 18

Split and Combined Treatments

Medicines cure diseases, but only doctors can cure patients.

—Carl Jung

Psychodynamic psychopharmacology is certainly appropriate for patients who only require pharmacotherapy. In other words, patients need not be classified as "treatment resistant" to benefit from this approach. However, when first-line pharmacotherapeutic approaches fail, concurrent pharmacotherapy and psychotherapy is a common approach and, in many cases, indicated. Combined treatments have been found to yield superior outcomes in patients who have treatment-resistant conditions, particularly depression (Cuijpers et al. 2009; Mintz 2022; Mintz and Belnap 2006; Pampallona et al. 2004). For these patients, the attitudes and skills that are practiced in psychodynamic psychopharmacology can not only deal with dyadic dynamics in ways that optimize outcomes but also facilitate the integration of the different treatments.

Approximately 20%–30% of patients prescribed psychiatric medications concurrently receive some form of psychotherapy (Olfson and Marcus 2009) or other mental health–related services. Historically, many psychiatrists provided this combined treatment. However, this is becoming less common as the field of psychiatry shifts away from psychotherapy practice (Mojtabai and Olfson 2008). As a result, most patients in psychotherapy are now in split treatment, with two (or more) providers tasked with attending to their mental health. Increasingly, such patients, who use not only significant psychiatric resources but also medical treatment resources, are part of integrated multidisciplinary care teams.

The move from dyadic to triadic to more complex systems of care, however, introduces a greater degree of complexity into the dynamics of treatment. Outcomes will be influenced not only by the psychology of the patient and quality of the prescriber–patient relationship (Krupnick et al. 1996) but also by different transferences to different members of the treatment team, creating the possibility for splitting and similar disruptive phenomena. Dynamic and often unconscious issues will play out between members of the treatment team that impact its effectiveness. Psychodynamic psychopharmacology offers practitioners tools for addressing the various complexities involved in working in triadic treatments, on treatment teams, and in systems of integrated care.

Integration and Nonintegration

Combining treatments does not necessarily make them integrated, just as split treatments may be highly integrated. Split versus combined and integrated versus nonintegrated are independent dimensions (Figure 18–1).

Split, Nonintegrated Care

It is not hard to envision how a split treatment might be nonintegrated. Such is the case when the prescriber and the psychotherapist each have their own treatment plans and targets, with little or no recognition of how their approaches may be similar, complementary, or discordant. In a worst-case scenario, such approaches may even be in direct opposition, as when a therapist is working to allow a patient to mobilize and release affect while the prescriber is aiming to help the patient suppress affect. The therapist wonders how she is going to help the patient whom she experiences to be in a medical fog. At the same time, the prescriber experiences the therapist as undoing his efforts to calm the patient and as undermining him when the patient reports that the therapist thinks she is overmedicated. In this case, the patient's prospects for a good recovery are, indeed, grim. When such significant interdisciplinary conflict arises, it is often wise to consider how the patient's intrapsychic dynamics or life history is being played out by the therapist, prescriber, and other members of the treatment team.

The adoption of a mind-body split may also be a strategy for dealing with interdisciplinary tensions and avoiding interdisciplinary conflict. As noted in Chapter 8, both the prescriber and the therapist may defensively avoid the gray zone at the intersection of meaning and medications. Psychotherapists may be reluctant to inquire too deeply into the meaning of medications because they do not want to be seen as impinging on the work of the pharmacotherapist, and vice versa. As a result, the important issue of the meaning of medications falls into the gap between the two disciplines (Mintz 2019). This may be particularly damaging when the patient's treatment resistance derives, in some measure, *from* medications, as discussed in Chapter 6.

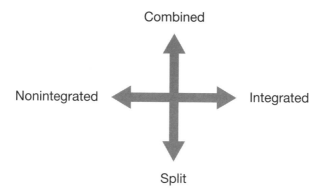

Figure 18–1.   Treatment combination and treatment integration.

Within psychoanalysis, such a split model is often advocated to protect the analytic function. In this view, a sharp distinction is drawn between the goals of pharmacotherapy and the goals of psychoanalytic treatment (Roose and Johannet 1998). In contrast to pharmacotherapy, which treats diseases, psychoanalysis treats subjects. Medication choices are therefore thought to be optimally guided by the nosology of DSM, based entirely on objective-descriptive criteria, in which issues of meaning or subjectivity play little role in medical decision making and "medication decisions should be based on the diagnostic system in the studies that established medication efficacy" (Roose and Johannet 1998, p. 612).

Combined, Nonintegrated Care

Combined treatment, with one psychiatrist who provides both psychother-apy and pharmacotherapy, may be integrated but is not necessarily so. One provider can easily wear these two hats in such a way that pharmacological and psychotherapeutic approaches are almost completely divorced. When the single prescriber-therapist has internalized a mind-body split, this may easily lead to a nonintegrated treatment; for example, the psychotherapeutic goals and pharmacotherapeutic treatment plan may conceivably be unre-lated, with the therapy addressing developmental goals while the pharmaco-therapy remains disease or symptom focused, with little reference to the larger psychotherapeutic goals.

It is not unusual for a mind-body split to be manifested in the structure of the treatment frame. This may be especially true for psychiatric trainees who are trying to master the complicated task of combining pharmacother-apy and psychotherapy and do so by dividing the treatment hour into a psy-chotherapy portion and a pharmacotherapy portion, both reflecting and facilitating a split in the work. Recent innovations in psychiatric coding that account for the minutes devoted to each task may further contribute to the impulse to divide the appointment into distinct parts. The patient, for example, complains to the prescriber-therapist: "Doc, you're killing me with this taper!" The psychiatrist responds to this as a medical statement in the context of a split model and responds: "Let's talk about that in the last 10 minutes of the hour, when we talk about medications." In this case, the doctor misses that the patient is making an interpersonal statement that has massive implications for the transference and the overall working relationship. Meaningful opportunities to explore the patient's experience of being harmed by the doctor are then lost, as well as opportunities for interpersonal repair. Optimally, statements about medications made in the context of a combined treatment will be heard by the prescriber-therapist as carrying important but possibly obscure meanings that address deeper concerns about the self and the transference to the prescriber-therapist.

The approach advocated in psychodynamic psychopharmacology does not endorse such a disease-centered view of the pharmacotherapeutic task. Rather, the patient-centered approach may be seen as being complemented by a "drug-centered" approach to prescribing that views medications not primarily as treating diseases but as having "distinctive drug-induced alterations to normal cognition, emotion and behaviour [that] can modify the manifestations of mental disorders independent of diagnosis or aetiological theory" (Yeomans et al. 2015, p. 229). The choice of medications may, in this perspective, be based on an understanding of the medication's likely effect on symptoms that are interfering with the patient's ability to achieve developmental goals (e.g., decreasing anxiety, decreasing expression of anger, helping the patient be less prone to feeling overwhelmed or impulsive, increasing energy or motivation).

Integration Between Pharmacotherapy and Psychotherapy

The integrated approach advocated in psychodynamic psychopharmacology is founded on very different assumptions than the principled mind-body split that sees pharmacotherapy and psychotherapy as distinct domains with different goals. Both treatment modes are seen primarily as addressing patients' developmental aims. Although pharmacotherapy certainly addresses symptoms, the ultimate goal of treatment is not symptom eradication (although this may happen). Rather, it is used to enhance patients' developmental capacities (e.g., agency, adaptability, resilience), facilitate their growth, and help them achieve their developmental aims. Addressing symptoms with medications serves these larger goals. To the extent that pharmacotherapy, like psychotherapy, is understood to serve the broader purpose of enhancing patients' developmental goals, integration between the two approaches is likely to be facilitated.

Combined, Integrated Treatment

In a combined, integrated treatment, with one psychiatric caregiver providing both psychotherapy and pharmacotherapy, psychiatric treatments function simultaneously at a biomedical and a psychosocial level. This is consistent with an evidence base that shows psychotherapy induces structural and functional changes in the brain (i.e., is a biological treatment) and that psychological and social factors are so crucial to the effect of medications that they may be understood to be primarily psychological treatments (Ankarberg and Falkenström 2008).

Viewing both modes of treatment as serving the goal of helping patients achieve their developmental aims lessens the potential for these treatments to be in overt conflict. However, the psychodynamic view also holds that people are complicated and almost always in conflict. Conflict will be introduced through the unconscious of the patient (and likely the prescriber). In a combined, integrated treatment, prescribers have established that their patients' relationship with pharmacological treatment will be a focus of psychotherapeutic exploration and will attend to evidence that symptoms or pharmacotherapy are serving defensive functions, medications are functioning as internal objects (Tutter 2006), transferences are directed toward medications, or the prescribing function is pulling for particular transferences, as described in Chapters 16 and 17.

Adhering to an integrated perspective, for example, the prescriber earlier whose patient stated, "Doc, you're killing me with this taper" would not hear this simply as a medical statement about symptoms but also as a remark on the state of the relationship and would be interested to explore further the patient's feeling that he is being harmed by the person who is supposed to care for him and the expectations associated with making such a statement.

Psychotherapist-prescribers should also be particularly attentive to the ways that they may be using medications as a defense against discomforting countertransference responses, acting out as a means of avoiding difficult aspects of the analytic function.

Ms. E (see Chapter 5) is a perfectionistic medical student who seeks treatment for depression, weight loss, and gastric pain. She has such a habitual need to please others that it has undermined her sense of self. In the first weeks of her treatment, she expresses a concern that her medications are making it harder for her to know what is truly her and what is medication.

For this reason, she has resisted her psychiatrist-psychotherapist's suggestion to discontinue Wellbutrin in favor of an antidepressant that is less likely to cause weight loss. In the first few months of treatment, her focus is on trying to identify her own desires and to develop a clearer sense of self, and her psychiatrist is comfortable with an approach that minimizes medication changes. Her gastric pain, which has not been found to be associated with any demonstrable pathology, persists, but Ms. E begins to gain weight.

Ms. E often reacts with intense emotional distress to changes in her somatic experience. Having read about somatization, she worries that her nonintegrated feelings will lead to real bodily damage and thus often feels an urgent need to fix something. Typically, they are able to trace this urgency back to earlier dynamics and her sense of having been damaged by misattuned caregiving, and Ms. E calms and feels contained. In one session, she complains of recent difficulty sleeping over several days, which she thinks needs urgent attention because she needs energy to study for her medical licensing examinations. Her prescriber-therapist suggests a mild hypnotic for short-term use. Ms. E declines the offer, citing her concern that medications are potentially alienating, and her urgency escalates.

Because the prescriber-therapist takes concrete action in prescribing, the prescribing function renders the therapist vulnerable to acting out disguised as therapeutic action. When the prescriber-therapist uses medications as a defense against distressing feelings evoked by the close encounter with the patient, it is particularly important to detect such enactments because there is a risk that they confirm for the patient, at least unconsciously, her deepest fears about her own intolerability.

In retrospect, the prescriber-therapist misunderstood Ms. E's primary aims in that moment. As her therapist, she counts on him to make sense of her experience and to help her know herself better. She values this over short-term symptomatic relief. Furthermore, she is working on an old developmental issue related to her experience of her family (and, subsequently, herself) as intolerant of her ordinary humanity. In the prescriber's offer of a prescription, Ms. E experiences a terrifying replication of her family's inability to accept her with her negative feelings.

In such cases, fortunately, therapists listen carefully for transference implications of their patient's speech. If patients experience their prescriber-therapist as acting out and voice this, the provider should consider how the patient is right because the patient may be offering helpful supervision. If therapist-prescribers engage defensively in a therapeutic misalliance and their patient is not consciously aware of this, the patient may still communicate this through associations (Langs 1975).

Ms. E's prescriber-therapist knows something is awry because Ms. E is much more anxious and hopeless in this session and the next, but he does not at first understand why. In her associations, she speaks of her family's insistence that one cannot complain until every remedy is attempted, of the counter-productive effects of her school's wellness curriculum, and of related topics that eventually highlight how she has experienced his offer of a prescription as trying to stop her from complaining and giving up on the effort to accept and understand her as she is. He is able to see how she is right, how her in-voking the medical licensing exam escalated his own anxiety (he, who is not so far from that experience himself), leading to a failure of containment. By interpreting her anxiety, he takes responsibility for his part in enacting a dis-tressing family dynamic. Her anxiety decreases not only because the alliance is restored but also because she experiences her doctor's nondefensive rec-ognition of his fallibility as increased permission for her own.

Although therapist-prescribers may strive not to engage in acting out, it is realistic to expect that unconscious impulses will play out beyond their awareness or control. As such, they must remain open to this possibility so as to become aware of entering into an enactment, with the goal of engaging its meaning, effecting needed repair in the therapeutic relationship, and re-turning to a state of true alliance (Plakun 2009). Getting into, detecting, and repairing such enactments often leads to better outcomes than would have happened without becoming involved in an enactment (Plakun 1998; Safran and Muran 2000).

Triadic Treatment and the Triadic Alliance

In the treatment dyad, the alliance is a key factor in determining treatment outcome, both for psychotherapy (Martin et al. 2000; Norcross 2002) and for pharmacotherapy (Krupnick et al. 1996). When moving from a dyadic to a triadic relationship, with two treaters and a patient, alliance (Kahn 1991) is a similarly important achievement. At the most basic level, a triadic alliance hinges on a negotiated or shared understanding of treatment goals that, in turn, is founded on recognizing that there will be a level of communication between treaters. Healthier patients may be able to serve as the conduit of in-formation about treatment goals and to alert the treatment team if there is some important incongruity between treaters. In general, however, treat-ment-resistant patients for whom psychodynamic psychopharmacology was developed will present with complicated dynamics that can easily promote splits in the treatment that reflect splits in their own inner world. In this case, patients may present themselves very differently to different treaters, show-ing different strengths and vulnerabilities and naming different struggles. Such patients, who often experience caregivers as starkly good or bad, may also generate splits by trying to make one treater into an ally against the other. Experiencing treaters through the lens of their persecutory inner world, they provide distorted reports about one treater (typically the "bad" one) to the other treater, creating an impression of conflict that may in turn generate real conflict.

Integration of care in split treatments begins with the establishment of an integrated treatment frame. As noted in Chapter 16, prescribers in the engagement phase of treatment focus on patients' life goals and then negotiate an approach that serves the patients' developmental goals. Often, this automatically establishes some synergy with the psychotherapy, which is likely also to be focused on the patients' broader developmental aims. Prescribers may want to facilitate integration by placing the pharmacotherapy in the service of the psychotherapy, particularly when the patient believes she is involved in important work, when the prescriber and patient are part of an explicit team, or when the patient is involved in a more comprehensive treatment such as a residential program, day treatment program, or intensive outpatient program.

If Mr. V (see Chapters 16 and 17) had been in psychotherapy or starting psychotherapy concurrently with pharmacotherapy, Dr. D would probably have concluded the first session somewhat differently. In addition to educating the patient about a psychodynamic approach that attends to meaning in pharmacotherapy and emphasizes a developmental perspective, she might also have negotiated an approach that puts the patient's learning and growth at the forefront. In such cases, prescribers may even make pharmacotherapy subservient to the psychotherapy, particularly if there is a close working relationship or team approach to the patients' care.

> Dr. D: Another thing that might be different from what you are used to with your previous prescribers is that I think of myself as prescribing, as I said, not to eliminate your symptoms, although that may happen, but to put you in the best place possible to maximize your gains in therapy. This may mean allowing you to still have enough anxiety that you can tell where the real problems are. For example, with your anxiety, it could take 10 mg of Klonopin to eliminate your anxiety completely. Now you may have no anxiety, but you won't remember a thing about what you worked on in your therapy.

When pharmacotherapy is aimed at supporting patients' capacity to grow through the optimal use of psychotherapy, therapists are much more likely to experience the pharmacotherapy as an adjunct to psychotherapy and thus to experience acting out with medications as a form of acting out in the transference. Because medications are explicitly intended to support patients' capacity to make use of therapy, problems with the optimal use of medications can be felt by the psychotherapist as treatment-interfering behaviors and manifestations of transference. The therapist may say to the patient, for example, "I've been curious about why you haven't been taking your [medication], given that Dr. Z is prescribing it to help you bear, among other things, the feelings that come up in therapy that make you shut down. It makes me wonder if your not taking the [medication] is a way of expressing ambivalence about deepening your work with me." In an integrated frame in which medications explicitly support psychotherapy, it becomes easier for the work of psychotherapy reciprocally to support the work of pharmacotherapy.

Communication Between Treaters: When and What To Communicate

Treatment integration between a psychotherapist and pharmacotherapist presumes a level of communication between treaters. The level of communication necessitated may hinge, to some extent, on patients' level of integration. Patients who rely on splitting as a primary defense mechanism may, for example, require more frequent contact to prevent internal splits from taking root in the therapeutic team. Conversely, patients who are well integrated may be counted on to convey important information between treaters. Unfortunately, treatment-resistant patients are more likely to fit into the former category. For patients who are not well integrated, the degree of integration between treaters may be a helpful corrective. Team-based care that facilitates communication and integration may allow sources of treatment resistance to be more effectively addressed.

> Such was the case with Mr. U (Chapter 12). He had engaged in intensive psychotherapy in a residential setting. Although intending to use the supports offered in residential treatment to taper off of a benzodiazepine, he had begun to have panic attacks of increasing intensity, and his use of benzodiazepines increased instead. Initially, Mr. U denied any context for his panic attacks, but his psychiatrist's uncovering of a relationship between the end of therapy appointments, increased suicidality, and then panic revealed that unexpressed anger toward the therapist seemed to drive the suicidality and subsequent panic and that the benzodiazepines served the maladaptive function of allowing Mr. U to plan his suicide without becoming anxious.
>
> In this context, it is made clear to Mr. U that he needs to discuss his frustration with his therapist. The patient, his therapist, and the psychopharmacologist meet together to review this triadic dynamic in which the negative transference has been split out, biologized, and left to the psychopharmacologist to try to detoxify. They agree that further anxiolytics are not warranted at this time, and Mr. U's "treatment-resistant" anxiety remits once the negative transference has been identified and engaged in the therapy.

At the outset, it is helpful to negotiate a triadic alliance that includes the psychotherapist. If the prescriber has set as a goal optimizing the patient's capacity to use therapy, then the psychotherapist should be made aware of this so the therapist can feel that resistances to medications are also potential

Table 18–1.   When and what to communicate with the therapist

Major clinical concerns

Major revision in the understanding of the patient's difficulties

Changes in the treatment plan that have the potential to affect the other clinician's work

When there is disagreement between treaters

When the patient complains about one clinician to the other

When one treater makes an intervention that potentially encroaches on the role of the other

resistances to therapy. Given that neither the therapist nor the psychopharmacologist will see all of the transference implications of medications, communication between treaters may expose ways the treatment arrangement is allowing transference to be split off and disguised. So that medications do not fall into a zone of inattention, the pharmacotherapist will optimally authorize the psychotherapist to examine the meaning of medication. At the same time, the prescriber will seek authorization from the psychotherapist to offer the patient limited interpretations exposing unconscious resistances to the healthy use of medications. Of course, with established working pairs or on treatment teams, these agreements do not have to be negotiated anew with each patient.

Certain clinical circumstances call for brief interdisciplinary communication (Table 18–1). When interdisciplinary disagreements are apparent, treaters will optimally try to reestablish concordance and understand what induced the disagreement, whether it is a difference in formulation about the nature of the trouble and the patient's clinical need or an external manifestation of the patient's internal splits. In the same vein, when a patient complains about one treater to the other (Busch and Gould 1993), communication about this can help modulate potential splits.

Interdisciplinary communication is also important when one treater has made an intervention that potentially encroaches on the role of the other. This may occur when a psychotherapist makes a medication recommendation to a patient (e.g., suggesting more, less, or a different medication). Leaving such an observation to the patient to communicate to the prescriber is fertile ground for splits. By the same token, practitioners of psychodynamic psychopharmacology are mindful not to interpret in such a way that establishes an alternate therapy. This can be done, first, by only addressing dynamics that are interfering with the healthy use of medication, and second, by letting the therapist know the content of an interpretation made to the patient so that formulations can be calibrated and the therapist is alerted to dynamics that may have been disguised or split off into pharmacotherapy. Ending interpretations to patients with the phrase "and I think you should talk to your therapist about this" serves as a reminder that deeper explorations are the purview of the therapist while also increasing the likelihood that patients will integrate medication issues into the therapy.

Key Points

- Combined psychotherapy and pharmacotherapy, administered by a single provider, can still be nonintegrated.

- Medications may be used by prescribers as a defense against discomforting countertransference responses and can be used in ways that undercut the tasks of psychotherapy.

- In split treatments, avoidance of overlapping zones of responsibility (i.e., the meaning of pharmacotherapy) may lead this issue to be neglected by all treaters, sometimes with serious consequences.

- Attention to goal concordance and an integrated treatment frame may minimize obstructive effects of splitting and foster a triadic treatment alliance.

- Periodic communication between psychiatric caregivers, particularly in the context of major changes in the patient or treatment or instances of potential conflict between treaters, promotes the integration of care.

References

Ankarberg P, Falkenström F: Treatment of depression with antidepressants is primarily a psychological treatment. Psychotherapy (Chic) 45(3):329–339, 2008 22122494

Busch FN, Gould E: Treatment by a psychotherapist and a psychopharmacologist: transference and countertransference issues. Hosp Community Psychiatry 44(8):772–774, 1993 8375839

Cuijpers P, van Straten A, Warmerdam L, et al: Psychotherapy versus the combination of psychotherapy and pharmacotherapy in the treatment of depression: a meta-analysis. Depress Anxiety 26(3):279–288, 2009 19031487

Kahn DA: Medication consultation and split treatment during psychotherapy. J Am Acad Psychoanal 19(1):84–98, 1991 1676395

Krupnick JL, Sotsky SM, Simmens S, et al: The role of the therapeutic alliance in psychotherapy and pharmacotherapy outcome: findings in the National Institute of

Mental Health Treatment of Depression Collaborative Research Program. J Consult Clin Psychol 64(3):532–539, 1996 8698947

Langs RJ: Therapeutic misalliances. Int J Psychoanal Psychother 4:77–105, 1975 1158612

Martin DJ, Garske JP, Davis MK: Relation of the therapeutic alliance with outcome and other variables: a meta-analytic review. J Consult Clin Psychol 68(3):438–450, 2000 10883561

Mintz D: Recovery from childhood psychiatric treatment: addressing the meaning of medications. Psychodyn Psychiatry 47(3):235–256, 2019 31448987

Mintz D: Combining medications and psychotherapy, in Textbook of Psychotherapeutic Treatments, 2nd Edition. Edited by Gabbard GO. Washington, DC, American Psychiatric Association Publishing, 2022

Mintz D, Belnap B: A view from Riggs—treatment resistance and patient authority, III: what is psychodynamic psychopharmacology? An approach to pharmacologic treatment resistance. J Am Acad Psychoanal Dyn Psychiatry 34(4):581–601, 2006

Mojtabai R, Olfson M: National trends in psychotherapy by office-based psychiatrists. Arch Gen Psychiatry 65(8):962–970, 2008 18678801

Norcross JC: Psychotherapy Relationships That Work: Therapist Contributions and Responsiveness to Patients. New York, Oxford University Press, 2002

Olfson M, Marcus SC: National patterns in antidepressant medication treatment. Arch Gen Psychiatry 66(8):848–856, 2009 19652124

Pampallona S, Bollini P, Tibaldi G, et al: Combined pharmacotherapy and psychological treatment for depression: a systematic review. Arch Gen Psychiatry 61(7):714–719, 2004 15237083

Plakun EM: Enactment and the treatment of abuse survivors. Harv Rev Psychiatry 5(6):318–325, 1998 9559350

Plakun EM: A view from Riggs—treatment resistance and patient authority, XI: an alliance based intervention for suicide. J Am Acad Psychoanal Dyn Psychiatry 37(3):539–560, 2009 19764850

Roose SP, Johannet CM: Medication and psychoanalysis: treatments in conflict. Psychoanal Inq 18(5):606–620, 1998

Safran JD, Muran JC: Negotiating the Therapeutic Alliance: A Relational Treatment Guide. New York, Guilford, 2000

Tutter A: Medication as object. J Am Psychoanal Assoc 54(3):781–804, 2006 17009655

Yeomans D, Moncrieff J, Huws R: Drug-centred psychopharmacology: a nondiagnostic framework for drug treatment. BJPsych Adv 21(4):229–236, 2015

CHAPTER 19

Psychodynamic Psychopharmacology and Integrated Care

*It is deeply satisfying to all mankind that many ailments, once danger-
ous, mysterious and worrying, offer the therapist of today wonderful
opportunities for the exercise of his skill; but with recalcitrant distress,
one might almost say recalcitrant patients, treatments tend, as ever, to
become desperate and to be used increasingly in the service of hatred
as well as love; to deaden, placate and silence, as well as to vivify. In
medical psychology the need for the therapist steadily to examine his
motives has long been recognized as a necessary, if painful, safeguard
against undue obtrusions from unconscious forces in treatment.... The
help of another in the review of one's unconscious processes is a much
better safeguard.... The temptation to conceal from ourselves and our
patients increasing hatred behind frantic goodness is the greater the
more worried we become. Perhaps we need to remind ourselves regularly that the word "worried" has two meanings, and that if the patient
worries us too savagely, friendly objectivity is difficult or impossible to
maintain.*

—Tom Main, "The Ailment" (1957)

Before the "decade of the brain," combined treatment with a psychiatrist-
therapist was a basic treatment model for patients who were receiving pharmacotherapy. Over the past three decades, however, practice patterns have
shifted dramatically. Meanwhile, the demand for mental health services has
escalated (Jorm et al. 2017) as the prevalence of psychiatric illness in the
United States appears to increase (Kessler et al. 2005). To enhance access to
and quality of care while limiting costs, models of integrated care have more

recently been promoted. *Integrated care*, according to the American Psychiatric Association (2021), "is a general term for any attempt to fully or partially blend behavioral health services with general and/or specialty medical services." Systematic reviews of integrated care models suggest improved outcomes in primary care patients and diverse populations and across a range of psychiatric illnesses (Jacob et al. 2012; Thota et al. 2012; Woltmann et al. 2012).

The Collaborative Care Model

In the collaborative care model (a particular model for providing integrated care) promoted by the American Psychiatric Association, "the Collaborative Care team is led by a primary care provider…and includes behavioral health care managers, psychiatrists, and frequently other mental health professionals *all empowered to work at the top of their license.* The team implements a measurement-guided care plan based on evidence-based practice" (American Psychiatric Association 2021, emphasis added).

This description of the collaborative care model, however, raises important questions from the perspective of psychodynamic psychopharmacology. One question pertains to goal setting. An aspect of the collaborative care model is a patient-centered perspective that emphasizes the importance of patient goals in the treatment plan. In this sense, psychodynamic psychopharmacology is a natural fit with the collaborative care model (Table 19–1). It provides psychiatric prescribers with the knowledge, skills, and attitudes necessary to explore and articulate patients' goals for treatment, often in a way that goes beyond mere symptom relief and more closely matches patients' more fundamental goals. In practice, however, biomedically focused prescribers may be pushed by the measurement tools that are available and familiar to set narrower, symptom-focused goals that are only tangentially related to patients' developmental aims. Mobilizing the skills of psychodynamic psychopharmacology facilitates the identification and incorporation of patients' goals into the treatment plan, helps elucidate how symptoms function to interfere with developmental goals, and provides an antidote to such reductionistic pressures while empowering patients to seek relief not only from symptoms but also from maladaptive patterns that put them at risk for relapse.

Furthermore, collaborative care models that empower mental health professionals to "work at the top of their licenses" raise the important question of what that means. Seen through a more biomedically reductionistic lens, the implication, ostensibly, is that whereas psychiatrists are licensed to prescribe, social workers and psychologists are not, so psychiatrists should focus their efforts on expert prescribing and leave the psychotherapeutic task to

Table 19–1. Psychodynamic psychopharmacology and collaborative care

Essential elements of collaborative care	Clinical tasks	Adding a psychodynamic psychopharmacology perspective
Patient-centered team care	Medical and mental health providers working at the top of their licenses	Recognition that the top of the psychiatric license involves using psychodynamic understandings and psychotherapeutic skills
	Collaboration using shared care plans that incorporate patient goals	Psychodynamic focus facilitates identification of patient-centered goals
Population-based care	Identification of patients who have not improved	Psychodynamic psychopharmacology developed to address needs of patients who have not improved
	Mental health specialists provide caseload-focused consultation, not just ad hoc advice	Caseload-focused consultation addresses individual and systems dynamics affecting outcomes
Measurement-based treatment to target	Each patient's treatment plan clearly articulates personal goals and clinical outcomes and is routinely measured by evidence-based tools	Psychodynamic focus ensures that measurements do not detract from patient-centeredness
	Treatments are actively changed if patients are not showing improvement as expected until the clinical goals are achieved	Treatments can include simple psychotherapeutic interventions under psychiatric guidance
Evidence-based care	Focus on provision of evidence-based care	Integrates evidence about *how* to prescribe, not just *what* to prescribe
Accountable care	Improved outcomes = improved reimbursement	More patient-focused and psychologically attuned care, attending to all the evidence bases, leads to better outcomes

less trained mental health professionals. In this view, prescribers serve a primarily biomedical function, providing psychopharmacological expertise that is beyond the ordinary capacity of primary care providers; the main tasks of the psychiatric consultant are to make accurate DSM diagnoses and provide recommendations for expert pharmacotherapy. Although primary care providers and their patients certainly may benefit from such an arrangement, they may also be deprived of the potential benefits of other aspects of psychiatric expertise.

Psychiatrists may be differentiated from other psychiatric prescribers, such as physician assistants and nurse practitioners, because psychiatrists receive extensive training in both psychotherapy and psychopharmacotherapy and in the integration of the two modalities. Therefore, the "top" of the psychiatric license naturally involves blending psychotherapeutic skills (including formulation) with psychopharmacological treatment. In the context of collaborative care, this means the consulting psychiatrist not only brings expertise about diagnosis and prescribing but also provides critical guidance about psychosocial, psychodynamic, and psychotherapeutic aspects of care.

The Disturbed and Disturbing Patient in the Treatment System

Such integrated skills are deeply needed in the primary care setting. The patients for whom psychodynamic psychopharmacology was developed are complex and often struggle with comorbid pathologies. Medical practices are filled with such patients, for whom medical need and emotional need are inextricably blurred and the degree of need outstrips the available resources for care. These patients, who may not have words for their feelings, often experience undifferentiated psychic distress as a bodily experience. They may struggle with medical care at various levels. Interpersonally, such patients often have complicated relationships with caregiving and are often quite ambivalent about their caregivers, treatment, or illness. Treatment seeking, for these patients, may serve multiple complex agendas. Manifestly, they seem to be seeking relief from symptoms. At a deeper level, however, other gratifications may actually be primary. As noted, they may primarily be seeking the experience of caregiving, and successful treatment of their symptoms would threaten their access to such caregiving. Alternately, they may be filled with rageful disappointment about failed caregiving and be motivated to thwart caregivers. These dynamics can sometimes be more unconsciously compelling to patients than the motivation to improve.

At the level of basic personality organization, these patients often rely on primitive defense mechanisms such as splitting and projective identification to manage overwhelming negative feelings such as helplessness, guilt, and shame. The use of such defenses often has profound implications for the systems in which these patients are treated, filling staff with bad feelings and creating interdisciplinary turmoil that can interfere with the well-being of staff and the effective delivery of care. To the extent that patients' somatic distress is largely a manifestation of unnamed and unaddressed emotional distress or a means of receiving care that is otherwise absent from their lives, medical interventions are likely to be largely ineffective or to have only short-lived benefit. Patients who unconsciously and defensively project their inner worlds into the outer world may force prescribers to experience states of emotional distress that they have not bargained on. With the skills inherent in psychodynamic psychopharmacology, the psychiatric consultant can enable the treatment team to integrate issues of meaning into an overall dynamic understanding of factors in the patient and the team that may interfere with optimal therapeutic care and contribute to treatment resistance.

An Integrated Perspective on Treatment Recommendations

A practitioner trained in psychotherapy and psychopharmacology who has buttressed these skills with added training in psychodynamic psychopharmacology is positioned not only to recommend specific medications based on an accurate diagnosis but also to recognize patients' diagnostic, developmental, and characterological features that would suggest a key role for psychotherapy. Mindful that developmental factors, such as defensive level (Joyce and Paykel 1989; Kronström et al. 2009; Scott et al. 1995), level of character organization (Skodol et al. 2011; Thase 1996), personality characteristics (Peselow et al. 1992), basic interpersonal positions (Bartholomew and Horowitz 1991), and fundamental beliefs and attitudes (Sullivan et al. 2003) have all been empirically demonstrated to affect pharmacotherapy outcomes, the most effective psychiatric consultant would be able to make an overall diagnosis (Balint 1969) that accounts for these factors. In turn, the consultant would be able to provide guidance about which patients would most benefit from psychotherapy in addition to medications and to suggest useful therapeutic targets for psychotherapy that are relevant to the patients' overall use (or misuse) of treatment.

Understanding the Dynamics of Treatment Resistance

Although population-based studies suggest a range of nonclinical patient characteristics that can adversely affect pharmacotherapy, many resistances to healthy use of pharmacotherapy are rooted in patients' unique psychology.

Psychiatric consultants trained in both psychotherapy and psychodynamic psychopharmacology are optimally positioned to elucidate such psychological resistances. In making an overall diagnosis, psychiatric consultants in collaborative care working at the top of their license are able to integrate their understanding of a patient's developmental history, basic relational paradigms, core conflicts, and adaptive efforts into a fuller understanding of the reasons that pharmacotherapy has failed to benefit the patient adequately. Furnished with this understanding, these consultants are then able to make recommendations regarding how to prescribe to optimize outcomes.

Importantly, in the primary care setting, the expertise of the psychodynamic psychopharmacologist does not apply only to the ways that patients' dynamics interfere with the healthy use of psychopharmacotherapy. Many of the dynamic resistances that emerge in relation to psychiatric medications tend also to emerge in relation to treatments for medical conditions. Consulting psychiatrists who are skilled in psychodynamic psychopharmacology may contribute helpfully to the medical care of patients by developing a guiding formulation that considers psychological contributors to nonadherence, poor response to medical treatments, and over- and misuse of medical treatment. Working with a sense of the overall diagnosis, they might observe that "insatiable dependence" (Groves 1978) underlies a patient's hateful and treatment-interfering attitudes and behaviors and offer recommendations that contain the distress of both the primary care provider and the patient. For a patient who is perceived to be a "manipulative help rejecter" (Groves 1978), the psychiatrist might, for example, recommend not only antidepressant medication and psychotherapy but also that the primary care provider share the patient's pessimism and lower expectations while setting a schedule of regular visits that contain the patient's dependency needs, minimizing unconscious pressure to manufacture new medical concerns that place unnecessary strains on both patient and doctor.

Teaching Ordinary Medical Psychotherapy

Psychodynamically savvy psychiatric consultants can also guide and educate medical providers and others on the integrated care team in the use of simple and effective psychological interventions that can enhance treatment outcomes. This is related to the model developed by Michael Balint in his work with primary care physicians in the United Kingdom who were treating "fat envelope" patients. Applying a psychodynamic understanding to these patients, Balint and colleagues fostered providers' capacity to offer "6-minute psychotherapy," which provides some containment of countertherapeutic dynamics, enhances outcomes, and decreases unnecessary treatment seeking. After elucidating the dynamics that foster treatment resistance, the consulting psychiatrist can help the primary care provider implement simple psychotherapeutic strategies to address hateful aspects of unnecessary care seeking. For example, rather than counterattacking with the "entitled demander," the provider can be guided to redirect the patient's entitlement into more effective patterns of help seeking and health management.

Managing Countertransference

Patients who are difficult to treat not only use limited medical resources because of their demands for care (whether expressed directly or through symptoms that require attention) and nonresponse to treatments but also place emotional demands on treaters. Such patients routinely thwart the narcissistic aspirations of treaters, tarnishing cherished fantasies that help treaters endure the arduous work of healing. Time and again, these patients show treaters the limits of their omnipotent striving to help and reveal the extent of their ignorance and impotence. Perhaps most painfully, such patients tax the kindness of their medical caregivers and confront them with the limits of their capacity to love. Furthermore, through projective identification, treaters are often forced, unconsciously, to bear disavowed feelings that have proven unbearable to the patients. When treaters are unaware that they are suffering on behalf of their patients, befuddlement about ego-dystonic reactions may be added to the negative feelings they are already bearing.

One consequence of this emotional demand is treater burnout. When heavy emotional demands resonate with lofty aspirations, treaters may be overcome with feelings of powerlessness and inadequacy. When patients evoke hateful counterreactions, guilt may then be added to the burdens the providers carry, as well as feelings of shame and exaggerated persecutory fears (e.g., of lawsuit or exposure) (Shapiro and Plakun 2008) that perpetuate a defensive practice of medicine. Treaters may react to hateful countertransferences with reaction formations (Maltsberger and Buie 1974), redoubling helpful efforts to cure and further draining both emotional and systems resources. Interventions, particularly as they become more extreme and irrational, may carry unconscious sadistic intent as patients are covertly punished by a regimen of intrusive, predictably low-yield tests and treatments.

When treatment begins to be dictated by countertransference, it is unlikely to be effective or efficient. This is, unfortunately, a common problem in primary care (as in psychiatry and other parts of medicine that deal with challenging patients). To deliver the most effective care and simultaneously be able to take care of themselves, primary care providers can benefit from consultation that helps them recognize, bear, and contain the countertransference reactions (Kjeldmand and Holmström 2008) that are impacting them, their patients, or both and are interfering with their delivery of effective care. Such consultation is at the heart of the psychodynamic psycho-pharmacologist's skillset.

With this skillset, consulting psychiatrists may help care providers on the treatment team understand their countertransference reactions. At a minimum, such recognition may minimize countertransference acting out, leading to improved care. If consultants can help other providers recognize the value of their countertransference feelings, then those feelings may also become less onerous. For example, when a provider is helped to understand that his feelings of helplessness and anger are a manifestation of an unbearable feeling with which his patient grapples on a daily basis, this understanding of underlying dynamics may help restore the provider's empathy (Treloar 2009). Furthermore, an ability to use countertransference reactions as data about patients may also help guide treatment interventions (Groves 1978).

Extremes of idealization and devaluation, as occur in splitting, are often difficult enough for individual practitioners to work with effectively. When such patients enter treatment systems, their primitive inner worlds are often projected into the outer world, which, in accordance with the patients' object representations, is frequently divided into those who are good and those who are bad. "Bad treaters" are reacted to with fear and hatred, are treated poorly, and in turn may feel fear or hatred toward the patient. "Good treaters" are treated with gratitude and, at least initially, evoke positive counter-transferences. Patients often turn to good treaters in search of allies against bad treaters and characterize the work with bad treaters, filtered through their own negative transferences, in ways that cultivate difference and mistrust in the treatment system. This is especially likely to happen when a patient's quest for allies against bad objects unconsciously exploits preexisting tensions in the system. The result is dysfunction in the treatment system, suffering among staff, and, potentially, gridlock in the patient's treatment because staff end up working at cross-purposes. These unfortunate events can also become fodder for burnout.

> Ms. W, a widowed woman in her early 50s, has recently switched to a new primary care practice after moving to be closer to her adult daughter. She has multiple medical issues, including obesity, chronic obstructive pulmonary disease, non-insulin-dependent diabetes, osteoarthritis, lower back pain, and recurrent kidney stones, as well as a history of depression. Her depression, although long-standing, worsened after the death of her husband from complications of alcoholism. She is enthusiastically grateful for the way she is treated in this new office, which she compares favorably with her previous doctor's office, which was more hurried, impersonal, and out of sync with trauma-informed principles. Between her gratitude and the story of her loss, she presents, initially at least, as a sympathetic character.

Over her first 6 months in the practice, Ms. W has not adequately responded to maximal dosages of several antidepressants nor to augmentation with an atypical antipsychotic. She has been referred for therapy and describes gratitude for her therapist, who is quite supportive and, she believes, really understands her. Her adherence with other treatment recommendations (nutritionist, respiratory care, adherence to prescribed medications) has, however, been less than optimal, which she attributes to her being too depressed to engage these parts of her life. Although still grateful for the care from her primary doctor and some of the nurses, she has begun to complain that some staff are brusque and insensitive to her loss and has tried to enlist the aid of some staff in educating the others about how to work with trauma (her loss) in a sensitive way. Some have made "helpful" interventions on her behalf, but these were not well received. The nutritionist and case manager have begun voicing increased frustration that the patient is rejecting the help they offer while complaining all the more vociferously about her symptoms. In the end, the "good" primary care provider and the therapist begin experiencing an increased demand from the system to treat Ms. W's depression so that she can participate more effectively in her own medical care. In this context, they consult the psychiatrist on the integrated care team.

If the consulting psychiatrist is skilled in assessing the ways that a patient's dynamics interact with treatments and treatment systems and is authorized by the systems to offer consultation aimed at the intersection of biological and psychosocial factors, teams can be restored to more optimal levels of function.

The psychiatrist, in accordance with the principles of psychodynamic psychopharmacology, routinely makes an assessment of the overall dynamics of treatment in addition to a DSM-focused psychodiagnostic assessment. He obtains a developmental history that illuminates expectable transference paradigms (and likely countertransference reactions) and directly assesses Ms. W's experience of care, including her feelings about illness, medications, and treaters. Through this process, he becomes aware of negative transferences directed toward some staff and of the likelihood that splitting dynamics have emerged on the treatment team. In addition to suggesting diagnostic interventions (adding borderline personality disorder) and pharmacotherapeutic interventions (recommending combined antidepressant therapy), he intervenes at the psychosocial level of treatment, educating the primary care provider and case manager about splitting dynamics. Although already well aware of splitting as a phenomenon, they have not appreciated that the tension in the staff was related to splitting.

With this consultation, the team works to mend their splits, and interdisciplinary and interpersonal tensions return to baseline levels. Staff are happier. Unfortunately, Ms. W is not, and several months later, the psychiatrist is consulted again. In this consultation, he ascertains that the team, who was experiencing Ms. W as manipulating them, closed ranks, and she began to think that her good treaters had given up on her. In essence, the disguised aggression that she previously directed at some members of the team, causing splits, has now been blocked by the team and redirected back at her. A second intervention is made in which the primary care doctor and team are 1) educated that splitting is not a conscious activity but an unconscious projection of the patient's inner world into the outer world and 2) offered a formulation to explain Ms. W's negative transferences and her need for allies. This seems to restore a measure of empathy for Ms. W and allows the team to work in a more integrated fashion. Team members are now, as a whole, more able to hold her responsible for her health behaviors, neither letting her off the hook because of her trauma nor angrily blaming her for her treatment resistance. In this context, her adherence to treatment recommendations improves.

Key Points

- Collaborative care models empowering providers "to work at the top of their licenses" optimally call for mobilization of all of the prescriber's skills, including psychotherapeutic skills and the ability to form an overall diagnosis that grasps patients more fully.

- Patients who seek unconsciously to address their unmet emotional needs through medical care may place excessive demands on their medical team.

- Primitively organized patients in medical care may project their inner worlds into the outer world, creating distress and discord in the medical care team.

- Consultants may use the skills of psychodynamic psychopharmacology to help medical teams address the psychological issues that are interfering with the optimal use of medical care and the disruptive systems effects of patients' relationship to care.

- Medical care providers may be taught rudimentary tools for basic and targeted psychotherapeutic interventions based on an understanding of patients' particular needs.

References

American Psychiatric Association: Integrated Care: Improving Access To Mental Health Services and the Overall Health of Patients. Washington, DC, American Psychiatric Association, 2021. Available at: https://www.psychiatry.org/psychiatrists/practice/professional-interests/integrated-care. Accessed June 2, 2021.
Balint E: The possibilities of patient-centered medicine. J R Coll Gen Pract 17(82):269–276, 1969 5770926

Bartholomew K, Horowitz LM: Attachment styles among young adults: a test of a four-category model. J Pers Soc Psychol 61(2):226–244, 1991 1920064

Groves JE: Taking care of the hateful patient. N Engl J Med 298(16):883–887, 1978 634331

Jacob V, Chattopadhyay SK, Sipe TA, et al: Economics of collaborative care for management of depressive disorders: a community guide systematic review. Am J Prev Med 42(5):539–549, 2012 22516496

Jorm AF, Patten SB, Brugha TS, et al: Has increased provision of treatment reduced the prevalence of common mental disorders? Review of the evidence from four countries. World Psychiatry 16(1):90–99, 2017 28127925

Joyce PR, Paykel ES: Predictors of drug response in depression. Arch Gen Psychiatry 46(1):89–99, 1989 2562916

Kessler RC, Demler O, Frank RG, et al: Prevalence and treatment of mental disorders, 1990 to 2003. N Engl J Med 352(24):2515–2523, 2005 15958807

Kjeldmand D, Holmström I: Balint groups as a means to increase job satisfaction and prevent burnout among general practitioners. Ann Fam Med 6(2):138–145, 2008 18332406

Kronström K, Salminen JK, Hietala J, et al: Does defense style or psychological mindedness predict treatment response in major depression? Depress Anxiety 26(7):689–695, 2009 19496102

Main TF: The ailment. Br J Med Psychol 30(3):129–145, 1957 13460203

Maltsberger JT, Buie DH: Countertransference hate in the treatment of suicidal patients. Arch Gen Psychiatry 30(5):625–633, 1974 4824197

Peselow ED, Robins CJ, Sanfilipo MP, et al: Sociotropy and autonomy: relationship to antidepressant drug treatment response and endogenous-nonendogenous dichotomy. J Abnorm Psychol 101(3):479–486, 1992 1386856

Scott J, Williams JM, Brittlebank A, et al: The relationship between premorbid neuroticism, cognitive dysfunction and persistence of depression: a 1-year follow-up. J Affect Disord 33(3):167–172, 1995 7790668

Shapiro ER, Plakun EM: Residential psychotherapeutic treatment: an intensive psychodynamic approach for patients with treatment-resistant disorders, in Textbook of Hospital Psychiatry. Edited by Sharfstein SS, Dickerson FB, Oldham JM, Washington, DC, American Psychiatric Publishing, 2008, pp. 285–297

Skodol AE, Grilo CM, Keyes KM, et al: Relationship of personality disorders to the course of major depressive disorder in a nationally representative sample. Am J Psychiatry 168(3):257–264, 2011 21245088

Sullivan MD, Katon WJ, Russo JE, et al: Patient beliefs predict response to paroxetine among primary care patients with dysthymia and minor depression. J Am Board Fam Pract 16(1):22–31, 2003 12583647

Thase ME: The role of Axis II comorbidity in the management of patients with treatment-resistant depression. Psychiatr Clin North Am 19(2):287–309, 1996 8827191

Thota AB, Sipe TA, Byard GJ, et al: Collaborative care to improve the management of depressive disorders: a community guide systematic review and meta-analysis. Am J Prev Med 42(5):525–538, 2012 22516495

Treloar AJ: Effectiveness of education programs in changing clinicians' attitudes toward treating borderline personality disorder. Psychiatr Serv 60(8):1128–1131, 2009 19648203

Woltmann E, Grogan-Kaylor A, Perron B, et al: Comparative effectiveness of collaborative chronic care models for mental health conditions across primary, specialty, and behavioral health care settings: systematic review and meta-analysis. Am J Psychiatry 169(8):790–804, 2012 22772364

Psychodynamic Psychopharmacology Self-Assessment Checklist

These self-assessment scales list some core behaviors recommended in the "Manual of Psychodynamic Psychopharmacology" in both the engagement (Table A–1) and maintenance (Table A–2) phases. The scales are intended to help learners track their overall progress in skill acquisition and to identify specific areas of strengths as well as skills for further development.

Table A–1: Engagement Phase

Table A–2: Maintenance Phase

Table A–1.   Psychodynamic psychopharmacology self-assessment checklist: engagement phase

Recommendation	1 = No (adopts primarily biomedical stance)	2 = Intermediate (recommendation partially or inconsistently implemented)	3 = Yes (implements recommendations of psychodynamic psychopharmacology)	Score
Demonstrate interest in the patient and not just symptoms.	Focuses discussion of medications around symptom presentation and reduction.		Prioritizes exploration of patient's values and developmental goals and the impact of illness on current life context.	——
Negotiate goals for treatment, including developmental aims.	Elicits goals oriented exclusively toward symptom reduction or remission.		Elicits goals oriented toward broader developmental aspirations and frames use of medication in the service of these goals.	——
Educate the patient about the impact of psychosocial factors on pharmacological outcomes.	Limits psychoeducation to the benefits and side effects of medications.		Discusses evidence base for the role of placebo, patient authority, motivation to change, therapeutic alliance, and other relevant evidence-based factors supporting good outcomes.	——
Discuss realistic limitations of pharmacotherapy without conveying hopelessness.	Talks as though all healing power rests in medicine and overpromises medical potency.		Discusses realistic limitations of pharmacotherapy and identifies hopefulness in leveraging the patient's authority.	——

Table A–1. Psychodynamic psychopharmacology self-assessment checklist: engagement phase *(continued)*

Recommendation	1 = No (adopts primarily biomedical stance)	2 = Intermediate (recommendation partially or inconsistently implemented)	3 = Yes (implements recommendations of psychodynamic psychopharmacology)	Score
In assessment note, include a formulation of the meaning of medication and potential sources of resistance.	Does not recognize psychosocial factors in the assessment, which is limited to diagnosis and somatic treatment options.		If there is a history of treatment resistance, assesses likely sources, including ambivalence about medications and illness, defenses at play, and potential negative transferences.	____
Obtain a developmental history that includes basic relational paradigms.	Limits developmental history to demographic data and substance use.		Elicits a developmental history that includes a focus on experiences with caregivers and authority and identifies basic and/or recurring relational patterns.	____
Explore experiences with and attitudes toward taking medication.	Does not ask about experiences with and attitudes toward taking medications.		Asks specifically about feelings toward and experiences of taking medication. Names potential anxieties about taking medications.	____

Table A–1.   Psychodynamic psychopharmacology self-assessment checklist: engagement phase *(continued)*

Recommendation	1 = No (adopts primarily biomedical stance)	2 = Intermediate (recommendation partially or inconsistently implemented)	3 = Yes (implements recommendations of psychodynamic psychopharmacology)	Score
Inquire about relationships with past psychiatric providers, including issues of autonomy and control.	Does not inquire about relationships with past psychiatric providers.		Asks specifically about patient's feelings toward and experiences with past providers and the mental health system. Names potential anxieties about the prescriber–patient relationship.	——
Explore ambivalence about illness, including what the patient might lose if treatment works.	Neglects patient's ambivalence about illness in initial evaluation.		Explores patient's fantasies about how medication may change his/her life, including concerns about what might be lost.	——
Name potential sources of resistance and include ongoing exploration of these sources in the negotiated alliance.	Neglects potential dynamic sources of treatment resistance and maintains a biomedical focus on the value of medications, with minimal attention to negative feelings about treatment.		Notes potential resistances, including feelings about medications, health, and medical authority, and recommends continued attention to these issues.	——

Table A–1.   Psychodynamic psychopharmacology self-assessment checklist: engagement phase *(continued)*

Recommendation	1 = No (adopts primarily biomedical stance)	2 = Intermediate (recommendation partially or inconsistently implemented)	3 = Yes (implements recommendations of psychodynamic psychopharmacology)	Score
Negotiate a treatment alliance that authorizes the patient and acknowledges the role of meaning in pharmacotherapy.	Interactional style emphasizes prescriber's authority and expertise.		Names patient's attitudes and engagement as important for optimal outcomes.	___
Educate the patient about the importance of noticing and working through problems in the alliance.	Adopts a paternalistic style that does not invite engagement about prescriber decisions and the state of the alliance.		Explicitly authorizes patient to engage prescriber about problems in the alliance. Patient is asked for his/her feelings about the initial engagement.	___
Involve patient in shared decision making that acknowledges patient's multilayered interests in treatment.	Makes medication recommendations from the position of medical expertise, with little exploration of patient wishes or offering of choices.		Elicits patient preferences, recognizing how patient preferences impact treatment outcomes.	___
			Total score	___

Table A–2.   Psychodynamic psychopharmacology self-assessment checklist: maintenance phase

Recommendation	1 = No (adopts primarily biomedical stance)	2 = Intermediate (recommendation partially or inconsistently implemented)	3 = Yes (implements recommendations of psychodynamic psychopharmacology)	Score
Adopt evidence-based prescriber practices that support positive outcomes to patient preferences.	Restricts evidence-based prescribing to the biomedical evidence base. Does not attend to psychosocial evidence or consider patient's psychology in adopting a clinical stance.		Uses evidence-based prescribing practices. Tailors stance (e.g., degree of warmth, investment, empathy) based on assessment of interpersonal preferences.	___
Consider meanings of medication changes and requests from the patient and prescriber.	Does not treat medication changes as having interpersonal meaning.		Explores interpersonal meanings of suggested medication changes on the part of both prescriber and patient.	___
Differentiate "problems of illness" from "problems of living"; find meaning in feelings.	Treats bad feelings as if they are only pathological and do not carry important information about current life troubles. Supports only biomedical solutions in ways that leave developmental opportunities unaddressed.		Explores the nature of dysphoric affects, including antecedents of bad feelings. Recognizes signal functions of those feelings and developmental opportunities.	___

Table A–2. Psychodynamic psychopharmacology self-assessment checklist: maintenance phase *(continued)*

Recommendation	1 = No (adopts primarily biomedical stance)	2 = Intermediate (recommendation partially or inconsistently implemented)	3 = Yes (implements recommendations of psychodynamic psychopharmacology)	Score
Explore evidence of ambivalence and offer tentative interpretations.	Prescribes as if the patient has no ambivalence. Does not inquire about or explore evidence of ambivalence.		Highlights ambivalence about pharmacotherapy as demonstrated behaviorally and verbally. Offers tentative interpretations to develop perspective on conflict.	___
Identify and name secondary gains that may promote treatment resistance.	Does not consider how the patient experiences psychological and interpersonal benefits of illness that complicate recovery.		Names overts and covert benefits to illness that could contribute to ambivalence.	___
Help translate communicative functions of symptoms.	Treats patient's symptoms simply as meaningless manifestations of aberrant biology and not as potential communications of unexpressed feelings.		Explores and names ways that symptoms may say something that patient cannot put into words (e.g., expressions of anger, fears of losing doctor).	___

Table A–2.   Psychodynamic psychopharmacology self-assessment checklist: maintenance phase *(continued)*

Recommendation	1 = No (adopts primarily biomedical stance)	2 = Intermediate (recommendation partially or inconsistently implemented)	3 = Yes (implements recommendations of psychodynamic psychopharmacology)	Score
Examine discrepancies between competing wishes, goals, and values while maintaining neutrality.	Maintains a symptom focus, not attending to resistances to treatment and how they relate to patient's broader developmental goals. Decides for patient which version of health patient should choose.		Highlights resistances to medications, prescribers, and health and considers the function of these resistances in light of broader developmental aims.	——
Recognize psychological defensive functions of symptoms while maintaining a nonjudgmental, interested, and curious stance.	Treats symptoms simply as meaningless manifestations of aberrant biology and not as potential solutions to inner conflict and/or presumes patient can and should simply stop using symptoms as solutions.		Listens for evidence that symptoms serve defensive functions. Recognizes importance of defenses and addresses underlying need for them. When needed, suggests medications may be more helpful if defensive uses are addressed in psychotherapy.	——
Listen for ways that problems in the alliance may negatively impact treatment.	Addresses problems with pharmacotherapy (side effects, nonresponse, nonadherence) only biomedically (e.g., changing prescriptions) without consideration of issues in the alliance.		Inquires about ways that side effects, nonadherence, nonresponse, and other complaints about medications may reflect a problem in the alliance.	——

Table A–2. Psychodynamic psychopharmacology self-assessment checklist: maintenance phase *(continued)*

Recommendation	1 = No (adopts primarily biomedical stance)	2 = Intermediate (recommendation partially or inconsistently implemented)	3 = Yes (implements recommendations of psychodynamic psychopharmacology)	Score
Address transference manifestations and work to differentiate the past from the present.	Does not consider how patient's past experience with caregivers will shape patient's response to prescriber.		Highlights how patient's past experiences may be transferred onto the current treatment situation, interfering with optimal outcomes.	___
Explore disempowering idealizing transferences.	Discusses medications as if patient only needs to wait to be healed.		Continues to express realistic humility about medications and importance of patient's role. Discusses instances in which idealizing transferences to doctor or medication promotes patient passivity.	___
Encourage help-seeking when medications have come to replace people.	Does not consider interpersonal consequences of reliance on substances rather than people for comfort and containment.		Highlights interpersonal consequences of use of medications rather than relationships for comfort and self-regulation. Encourages use of people before medications.	___

Table A–2. Psychodynamic psychopharmacology self-assessment checklist: maintenance phase *(continued)*

Recommendation	1 = No (adopts primarily biomedical stance)	2 = Intermediate (recommendation partially or inconsistently implemented)	3 = Yes (implements recommendations of psychodynamic psychopharmacology)	Score
Focus on coping skills when patients have become deskilled by overreliance on medication.	Encourages use of medications for distress without recognizing possible internal resources for self-regulation or supporting development of more mature coping skills.		Identifies restricted coping due to reliance on medications. Supports use of coping skills (including, as needed, referral to psychotherapy). Tapers gradually at a rate that avoids overwhelming undeveloped coping skills.	——
Consider how the patient is right when negative transference is expressed.	Explains away complaints or becomes defensive. Assumes patient is simply distorting when he/she responds negatively to prescriber.		Considers how feedback from patient illuminates areas in which prescriber is functioning in ways that undermine working alliance.	——
			Total score	——

Glossary of Psychodynamic Concepts Relevant to the Practice of Pharmacotherapy

acting out

Defense mechanism wherein distressing feelings, thoughts, and impulses are discharged through action rather than represented mentally or in words. Of particular importance in pharmacotherapy is the tendency to take action with medications (e.g., overdoses or nonadherence) rather than experiencing ambivalent and distressing feelings.

alexithymia

Literally, "no words for feelings." Developed by Peter Sifneos and further explicated by Henry Krystal, Joyce McDougall, and others. Individuals experience emotions as diffuse states of emotional or physical arousal that they are unable to describe beyond very basic labels. They tend to have limited imaginal lives and are more likely to somatize distress and to experience substance abuse.

ambivalence

Pervasive characteristic of mental life whereby contradictory feelings and impulses coexist, such as might occur when patients want to be cured of depression but fear the loss of caregiving if they become well enough to care for themselves. Such patients might ask for medications but then repeatedly neglect to take them.

as-if personality

Personality style, initially described by the psychoanalyst Helen Deutsch, in which the person presents as manifestly making a good social adjustment that covers a profound sense of alienation from the self and a lack of authenticity. Motivations are dominated by a need to conform to the wishes and expectations of others. Also called "false-self" (Winnicott) and normopathy (McDougall). Patients have little or no sense of a genuine self, and medications may exacerbate confusion about what is real about them.

attachment style
Fundamental relationship paradigms, conditioned at least in part by the person's earliest relational experiences with caregiving and shaped by both the sense of self and sense of other as either positive or negative. Concept comes from attachment theory, initially developed from the work of John Bowlby. Medication responses tend to be more robust when there is a secure attachment (positive self and positive other). Dismissive attachment (positive self and negative other) tends to lead to issues with adherence and lack of benefit. Anxious-fearful attachments (negative self–negative other) may be nocebogenic (*See* nocebo effect).

autonomy
As defined by Aaron Beck, a personality style characterized by a drive for individual achievement and for interpersonal freedom and a tolerance of solitude. Linked to a higher response rate in patients who take antidepressants.

biopsychosocial
Model based on general systems theory that considers disease processes to manifest at multiple levels, including the biological (e.g., neurochemical alterations), psychological (e.g., distress, defenses, illness behaviors), and social (e.g., the sick role, stress in the family system, stigma). Perturbations at any level can affect the surrounding levels. The extent to which this happens depends on the severity of the perturbation and the premorbid stability of that level (e.g., patient does or does not have good social supports).

body ego
Sense of self and personal identity rooted in bodily experience. In psychoanalytic theory, the ego, or the "I," first emerges in a child's sense of bodily coherence. Patients whose sense of self-coherence is disrupted by psychosis may find medications especially threatening when they induce changes in bodily experience that cause the body to feel unfamiliar.

Cartesian dualism
Fundamental tenet of Descartes' philosophy that humans are composed of two distinct substances: body, which is physical and mechanistic, and mind, which is ephemeral, indivisible, and spiritual. The thinking of Descartes, the

17th century philosopher and mathematician, has been highly influential in the intellectual traditions of Western civilization. Dualistic metaphors have been ingrained in Western culture and language in ways that promote dualistic thinking in the approach to psychiatric illness.

chronification
Concept from the neurological literature on headache wherein overreliance on pharmacotherapy perpetuates headache, creating a vicious circle in which headache becomes chronic. In psychiatry, this may occur when overreliance on medications to contain psychic distress leads to worsening distress and greater need for medications. An example is a patient who so relies on medications to dull feelings of upset and of being overwhelmed that the patient loses other, healthier skills for managing affects and becomes more prone to feeling overwhelmed, leading to further reliance on medications.

compromise formation
When a conflicted wish or idea is repressed but finds expression in disguised form, such as a dream or symptom that serves as a compromise between the expression and repression of the wish. Defense mechanisms are another form of compromise formation. When symptoms serve as expression of a forbidden impulse, patients may be ambivalent about relinquishing them. Medication use may itself be symptomatic and serve as a compromise formation, such as when medications are used in a way to manage aggression. The patient takes medications to dull feelings of rage but takes them in a way that saps him of initiative. Thus, medications also implicate those who cannot tolerate his anger in his self-destruction while also directing the aggression toward the self through a self-destructive use of medications.

concordant countertransference
Form of countertransference first described by Heinrich Racker in which the treater experiences feelings that mirror those in the patient. For example, a patient who feels angry or helpless induces corresponding feelings in the treater. If not identified and managed, such countertransferences can introduce irrationality into the prescribing process. If identified, however, these experiences can become a source of empathy and understanding for the patient.

conflict
An essential feature of the human mind because competing agencies (id, ego, superego) and wishes are almost always in conflict (e.g., a wish for intimacy but fear of being hurt by or trapped in dependency). Anxiety is a common result of intrapsychic conflict, but many other defenses, more or less adap-

tive, are used unconsciously to keep such conflict out of awareness. In pharmacotherapy, patients are likely to experience conflicts about receiving psychiatric treatment and taking medications.

countertransference
Sometimes understood simply as the treater's emotional response to the patient. Alternatively understood as the treater's emotional response to the patient's transference. Viewed in this latter way, it can be seen as a tool for identifying and understanding aspects of the patient's unconscious. Attention to and curiosity about one's reactions becomes an important part of the work of psychiatric care providers, particularly with patients who are difficult to treat and evoke strong reactions. Unacknowledged countertransferences may lead prescribers to make medication decisions that are irrational.

defeating process
Conscious or unconscious effort to defeat the treatment, and thus the treater, usually in retaliation for a real or perceived injury, slight, or frustrated wish. Defeating processes may be one source of pharmacological treatment resistance.

defense
An unconscious psychological process intended to keep conflicted and distressing thoughts, feelings, and wishes out of conscious awareness. Defenses vary in the degree to which they recognize and adapt to reality. The degree to which they adversely impact the person depends on the maturity and the flexibility/adaptability of the defenses employed. When either medications or illness serve defensive functions, patients may unconsciously resist treatment.

denial
Unconsciously driven refusal to perceive and acknowledge aspects of reality to avoid distress that would be associated with acknowledging that reality. Regarded as a more primitive or immature defense mechanism because it involves a high degree of reality distortion. Commonly seen in substance abuse in a fixed and inflexible form and in psychotic disorders in which basic realities are simply denied. An example encountered in the context of pharmacotherapy is a patient with schizophrenia who reasons that by refusing antipsychotic medication, psychosis is thereby also negated.

dissociation
Defense against trauma or significant stress in which there is a consciously experienced separation from the environment (resulting in derealizations) or discontinuity in the sense of self (resulting in depersonalization, amnesia, or discontinuous identities).

ego
Psychological apparatus oriented toward reality that serves to moderate sexual and aggressive impulses in light of the demands of civilized society. Functions include perception, insight, and coherent sense of self.

ego-dystonic
Thoughts, feelings, or actions experienced as being incompatible with one's conscious wishes, motivations, values, and personal identity.

ego functions
Mental functions involved in a person's adaptation to reality, including perceiving self and the environment, use of memory, problem solving (finding compromise between competing demands of the id, superego, and reality), and affect regulation. Patients who rely heavily on medications to manage intense affect states may fail to develop more mature affective coping skills (*See* ego).

enactment
Reproduction, in the therapeutic relationship, of important relational paradigms from the patient's inner world. The patient's transference engages an important aspect of the treater's psychology in a way that induces the treater to respond emotionally and behaviorally in ways that actualize transference expectations. An unavoidable aspect of charged therapeutic relationships. Because prescribing is an action taken by clinicians within a complex and charged relationship, it may be particularly prone to becoming an enactment.

false-self
Concept associated with the work of psychoanalyst D.W. Winnicott. Although a prominent false-self may lead to feelings of emptiness, meaninglessness, and inauthenticity, all people probably have some aspect of a false-self in terms of our need to present ourselves in pleasing and agreeable ways to each other. A patient with a predominant false-self experience may present with vague feelings of depression that most likely will not respond well to medication and may also find that medications introduce further confusion as to what is authentic to the self (*See* as-if personality).

hostile dependency
Defensive relationship pattern in which one or both participants are dependent on the other but are motivated not to be aware of dependency. Instead of feeling need, the onus is shifted, and the person in question feels entitled to need-gratifying responses and anger at the other for their inadequacies or failings. Patients with such dynamics who feel some need for their health care providers may complain of being failed, whereby they attempt to hold the prescriber responsible through guilt.

immature defenses
Defenses may be assessed as more or less mature based on the extent to which they interfere with recognition of and appropriate reaction to reality. Immature (primitive) defenses that involve a greater degree of reality distortion are linked to worse outcomes with medications, particularly antidepressants.

inexact interpretation
Proposed by Edward Glover, an explanation of the patient's actions, motivations, and distress, often along biomedical lines, that contains enough truth that the patient can defensively seize on the explanation to avoid facing more distressing insights. An example is a patient with borderline personality disorder who is told that her interpersonally destructive acting out is related to her bipolar disorder. She seizes onto this explanation because it relieves her of guilty responsibility for her actions and locates the blame in an illness or the doctor who fails to contain the illness.

interpretation
Psychodynamic technique that involves putting into words the psychodynamic clinician's understanding of the patient's unconscious defenses and motives in the service of disrupting conscious, defensive everyday ways of self-understanding, increasing insight, and extending the patient's conscious agency. Interpretation of the patient's unconscious expectations of pharmacotherapy may help address sources of treatment resistance.

intrapsychic
Mental phenomena, including thoughts, feelings, impulses, and defensive operations, that arise primarily within the person's mind and pertain to the relationship to the self.

locus of control
Psychological variable relating to individuals' sense of how much they are in control of the conditions and outcomes of their lives. People with an *external* locus of control see their trajectories as determined largely by environmental

and interpersonal factors beyond their control. People with an *internal* locus of control tend to believe that they are ultimately in charge of their own destiny. Can shape pharmacotherapy outcome, with internal locus contributing to better outcomes with antidepressant pharmacotherapy.

manic defense

Defense against feelings of vulnerability, dependency, loss, and guilt. Such vulnerability is denied through a driven focus on activity that distracts from the more vulnerable feelings and a dismissive stance that denies the value of the needed object. The combination of driven activity and dismissiveness can be confused with hypomania but may be distinguished from it by identifying a defensive, distracting function served by the activity and by an absence of other features of bipolarity, such as a significantly decreased need for sleep.

narcissistic defenses

Defenses intended to protect one's self-esteem whereby idealized aspects of the self are preserved and limitations denied. Although protecting self-esteem is a universal concern, narcissistic defenses in the presence of a low or damaged self-esteem with predominant feelings of shame tend to promote compensatory grandiosity that is rigid and totalistic. Such patients may be inclined to reject medications, consciously or unconsciously, because medications imply a degree of need or lack. These patients, when depressed and depleted, may seek treatment, but if medications work and narcissistic defenses are reconstituted, they are motivated to stop medications.

negative identity

Reaction, described by Erik Erikson, of a person who is frustrated in the development of a cohesive and positive identity (typically as defined by familial or societal norms). Rather than experience inadequacy in relation to the ideal, the person embraces its opposite. Typical example is a delinquent child who appears to embrace his badness as a badge of honor rather than a mark of shame. Similar dynamics may play out with patients who embrace negative elements of the sick role.

neuroticism

Relatively stable personality factor marked by a degree of emotional instability and tendency toward worry, depression, self-doubt, and other dysphoric affects. Appears to be a negative prognostic factor for treatment with antidepressants.

nocebo effect
Inverse of the placebo effect. Occurs when conscious or unconscious expectations of harmful effects of treatment promote the development of harmful effects. Multiple lines of evidence suggest that experiences of powerlessness increase proneness to nocebo effects.

object relations
School of psychoanalytic thought positing that early relationships that are internalized (e.g., the belief that you are good and caring but I am bad and undeserving) form the basis of intrapsychic and interpersonal functioning. These internalized object relationships or relational paradigms become the model for experiencing self and other and color how the patient is likely to experience the treater and may also be mapped onto medications, which are then experienced as serving important emotional and interpersonal functions (e.g., comforting, controlling, punishing).

observing ego
Aspect of conscious mental functioning that allows individuals to step back from the pressing emotional and defensive demands of a situation and to reflect, impartially and reasonably, on their own mental activity and actions.

orality
In psychoanalytic theory, a style or focus on objects and activities that relate symbolically to the early feeding situation. The hunger and voraciousness that characterize people with strong oral fixations can be focused on food (as in binge-eating disorder), can manifest interpersonally (e.g., a consuming needfulness), can be channeled into a hunger for treatment, or can fuel a desire for medications, which symbolically gratify a need to incorporate something nutritious, good, and associated with loving care.

overall diagnosis
The idea, deriving from Michael Balint's work with complex medical patients, that a thorough diagnostic understanding of the patient includes not only a biomedical diagnosis but also an understanding of psychological factors involved in care seeking and unhelpful use of treatment.

primitive object relations
Object relations in which mental representations of the self and other are not integrated into complex forms that contain positive and negative aspects but rather are only fragmentary, for example, carrying only goodness or badness. Patients with predominantly primitive object relationships have an unstable sense of self and unstable relationships because they shift back

and forth from markedly disparate and unintegrated images of the self and other. Such patients typically rely on primitive defense mechanisms such as splitting and projective identification.

projection
Defense mechanism by which an unwanted aspect of the self is disavowed and then experienced as being a characteristic of another person or group. When undesirable qualities are projected onto prescribers (e.g., being only motivated by narcissistic concerns), the alliance may be weakened and resistances to treatment fortified.

projective identification
Defense mechanism in which the patient projects some unwanted aspect of the self onto another (e.g., spouse, therapist, prescriber) and then behaves in such a way as to induce the unwanted feeling in that person, who now serves as a container for the unwanted emotional experience. Relatively immature defense mechanism that differs from other defense mechanisms because it involves engaging another person in the action of the defense. Although often seen in patients with personality disorders, it may also be observed in families, couples, and group dynamics. In pharmacotherapy, one manifestation is a patient who is intolerant of feelings of powerlessness or helplessness. Consequently, she refuses to be constrained by the prescriber's recommendations, taking too little or too much medication. In this context, the prescriber comes to feel helpless.

psychological-mindedness
Mental capacity to reflect on the minds of others and on one's own mind, to be able to differentiate ideas and feelings from reality, and to consider the symbolic meaning of behavior.

psychotic anxiety
Anxiety in persons with or near psychosis in response to de-differentiation, fusion, or disintegration that is experienced as free-floating and an intensely distressing threat of the loss of self. Delusional fixations are one possible outcome because patients strive to find a concrete explanation for their sense that something is dangerously wrong.

reaction formation
Defense mechanism in which an unacceptable thought, feeling, or impulse is denied and replaced in conscious awareness with its opposite. Examples in pharmacotherapy include a patient who is unconsciously enraged at caregiving but transforms it into obsequiousness, or a mental health clinician

who feels persecuted by a patient's chronic suicidal threats and transforms that anger into a benevolent and self-sacrificing therapeutic zeal.

reflective functioning
See psychological-mindedness.

resistance
Efforts, generally unconscious, made by patients to prevent their disavowed unconscious mental content from being brought to conscious awareness in psychodynamic treatment. When medications or their meaning facilitate such disavowal, resistance may also manifest as resistance to the effects of medications or to withdrawal of countertherapeutic medications.

signal function
Idea that affects, particularly anxiety, serve to alert individuals to dangers, whether internal or external. In psychoanalysis, anxiety that occurs without a clear context often signals that a defended-against thought, feeling, or impulse is at risk of being expressed and brought to conscious awareness. In this sense, anxiety helps the patient and clinician know where to look to unearth important conflicts. Patients may use medications to blunt or obscure the signal functions of their affects, interfering with their ability to use affects as a guide.

splitting
Immature defense mechanism that is a prominent mode of defense in Cluster B personality pathology. Avoids ambiguity and conflict by casting the self and other in stark, black-and-white images that are experienced as either good or bad. These polarized images can shift rapidly so that one may be idealized in one moment but devalued in the next. Although such polarized idealization and devaluation can be extremely disruptive in treatment, splitting may be understood as an unconscious attempt to manage conflicted feelings in a manner that protects the unblemished positive images of people who are valued by the patient.

superego
Mental agency that holds the person's values and ideals. An overly harsh and self-critical superego can promote depression when directed at the self and alienation when directed toward others. A weak superego promotes impulsivity because constraints of ethics and propriety cannot counterbalance the drive for immediate gratification. Superego strength may factor into medication decisions because patients with superego deficits are more likely to misuse medications that induce pleasurable responses.

sociotropy
Personality style characterized by a strong need for social approval, anxiety about separation, and a drive to please others. Linked to a lower response rate to antidepressants.

somatization
Unconscious defensive process whereby psychological distress is displaced into the body and experienced as bodily symptoms, sparing the person from awareness of emotional distress.

symbolic equation
Primitive mode of thinking described by Hanna Segal that equates current objects with past objects rather than finding a resemblance between them. Psychological trauma can collapse boundaries between inner and outer worlds; things reminiscent of the trauma become the trauma itself. Medications, for example, may be experienced concretely as a sexual assault.

therapeutic alliance
Originally described by Elizabeth Zetzel, an aspect of the therapeutic relationship (which also includes the transference relationship and the real relationship) that forms when a bond develops between the patient and the clinician, and the reasonable and healthy strivings of the patient join with the clinician to find common cause and agency around the tasks and goals of treatment. Has been determined to play a significant role in the outcome of pharmacotherapy in depression and other psychiatric conditions.

transference
Unconscious mapping of early relational models (usually to primary attachment figures) onto people in the patient's present day, leading the patient to respond to these present-day figures with emotions and expectations from those prior relationships. Although transferences happen in everyday life, they have special significance in the clinical caregiving situation because they simultaneously reveal, in the here and now, aspects of the patient's unconscious, serve as vehicles for treatment (working through persisting early wishes and fears in the present), and become vehicles of resistance to therapy (*See* transference resistance). Transferences to the psychiatric prescriber or medication may further or hinder therapeutic outcomes.

transference resistance
Particular form of resistance in which the transference itself becomes the vehicle of resistance to insight. For example, a patient develops an erotic transference to his therapist and wants to present in such a way as to win the

therapist's love. Now he cannot consider revealing his darker and less attractive aspects and resolves to keep these important aspects of himself out of therapy; thereby, the transference becomes a resistance.

transitional objects
Comforting objects that occupy a position between inner and outer reality and between utter reliance on a parental figure and the capacity for self-soothing. Although real physical objects, such as a teddy bear or blanket, they are also imbued by the person with emotional importance and experienced as largely under the person's control, which provides a sense of security. Medications may function for some adults as transitional objects, creating a feeling of security ("I can be calm as long as I have my lorazepam in my pocket") and a strong emotional attachment to the medication.

unconscious
Core tenet of psychoanalysis that a dynamic unconscious is created by the need to keep distressing and conflictual mental content out of awareness. The processes (i.e., defense mechanisms) whereby distressing content is kept out of awareness are also unconscious. These processes, at the same time, often allow unconscious content to be expressed in disguised form, so the unconscious is continually influencing the person's conscious mental life and behavior. Conscious awareness is only a small portion of mental life. Implication for pharmacotherapy is that unconscious factors are always impacting the patient's response to medications.

working alliance
See therapeutic alliance.

working relationship
See therapeutic alliance.

working through
Process in which unconscious patterns are repeatedly brought to conscious awareness, incrementally overcoming resistance to insight and then resistance to change.

Index

Page numbers printed in **boldface** type refer to tables and figures.